3 Minutes *to a*
Pain-Free Life

3 Minutes *to a* Pain-Free Life

The Groundbreaking Program for Total Body Pain Prevention and Rapid Relief

Joseph Weisberg, P.T., Ph.D., *and*

Heidi Shink

ATRIA BOOKS

New York   London   Toronto   Sydney

This publication contains the opinions and ideas of its authors. It is intended to provide
helpful and informative material on the subjects addressed in the publication. It is sold
with the understanding that the authors and publisher are not engaged in rendering medical,
health, or any other kind of personal professional services in the book. The reader should
consult his or her medical, health, or other competent professional before adopting any
of the suggestions in this book or drawing inferences from it.

The authors and publisher specifically disclaim all responsibility for any liability, loss,
or risk, personal or otherwise, which is incurred as a consequence, directly or indirectly,
of the use and application of any of the contents of this book.

ATRIA BOOKS
1230 Avenue of the Americas
New York, NY 10020

Copyright © 2005 by Joseph Weisberg, Ph.D. and Heidi Shink

ISBN 0-7434-7647-6 (alk. paper)

ATRIA BOOKS is a trademark of Simon & Schuster, Inc.

Manufactured in the United States of America

This book is dedicated to Stella Forer, whose immense love of life and laughter shows us that it is possible to age gracefully; and to the memory of Zipora Weisberg, whose kindness, insight, and brilliance continue to illuminate the lives of those she touched.

Acknowledgments

Writing this book was not a solitary experience. Many generous people contributed their time and talents throughout the process, creating an environment where the dream of bringing this work to fruition would become a reality.

Heidi and I would like to express our gratitude to our editor, Tracy Behar, for her instantaneous response to our work ("You had me with the title!"), unwavering commitment, and extraordinary vision that nurtured and shaped the book. We would also like to thank our agent, Matthew Guma, for his tireless efforts, innumerable ideas, and unending energy. Matthew Jones provided invaluable, unbiased, and expert legal advice on our journey toward publication. Christy Stoner put her considerable abilities to work to produce amazing illustrations. David Daigle pulled out all the (F) stops, photographing the therapeutic movements with unbelievable clarity and beauty. Robin Morrell organized the logistical framework that made my busy life manageable. Dr. Bernard Lender, president of Touro College, afforded me the flexibility to dedicate my time to writing. Drs. Bert Agus and Laura Jacobs and pharmacists Wendy Jones and Jodi Levine gave essential professional insights.

Our heartfelt appreciation extends to our models: Michele Cherry-Grace, Jabari Hearn, Angie Lee, Brendan O'Reilly, Michael Papadol, and Nathan Peitzmeier, who patiently endured hours of being positioned and prodded (while not stepping on the white backdrop) with enthusiasm and good humor. And the testimonial writers were gracious enough to make their private stories public, illuminating how individual battles with pain can be transformed into triumphs.

On a personal note, we'd like to thank an assortment of close friends and family who gave us emotional and practical help throughout the writing of the book. Dani Alpert, Michelle Rivera, Amy Ruskin, and Leah Stansbury were each there when needed most, whether to unblock writer's block, offer words of encouragement, or share the myriad emotions that came up while undertaking this project. Harlan Levine supplied a constant source of necessary levity through e-mail. Amy Utstein and Rebecca Raphael, both bristling with wonderful ideas, donated their expertise in preediting the proposal and book. Steve Utstein gave incredible word-processing tutorials, making the often treacherous technology a little less daunting. Denise Hammond tapped her formidable resources, ensuring that the photo shoot was balanced and complete. Jonnie Stansbury offered helpful direction and wise counsel. Aunty and Uncle Rabin not only introduced us to each other, but prepared the most delicious food before and after all of our late-night writing sessions. And GG, the first person to know that we were writing this book, believed in it fully when it was just a seedling of an idea.

Finally, Heidi's very special thanks goes to Simon and Vicki Shink for always being there with unconditional love, guidance, and support. And to Caitlin Stansbury, who inspired her to find creativity and courage on a daily basis. My deepest thanks goes to Arel, Yaron, Orah, and Yael Weisberg, who gave of themselves through unwavering advice, tolerance, and understanding. And especially to Rina Weisberg, whose complete devotion to the family and total support of my professional goals made it possible for me to write this book.

Contents

Part III: Special Circumstances

Introduction
by Heidi Shink

"Do you brush your teeth every day?" Those were the very first words that Dr. Weisberg said to me. Had I not been lying prone on his examination table in excruciating pain and almost completely immobile, I would have gotten up to make sure that the nameplate on his office door read "Physical Therapist" and not "Dentist." After all, I thought to myself, what on earth do my teeth have to do with my lower back? As it turned out, everything. Dr. Weisberg explained to me that he had developed a program that would do for my recurrent aches and pains what brushing and flossing did for my teeth. And it would take about the same amount of time to accomplish.

It seems inconceivable from today's perspective, but preventive dental care is a rather new concept. At the turn of the last century, the simple act of protecting and maintaining one's teeth daily was not part of life's routine. Consequently, it was common for people to begin losing their teeth as young as age 30; by age 50, many had none left in their mouths. At the time it was widely believed that human teeth were simply unable to last the span of a full life. We now know this to be totally erroneous. The truth is that the methods (or lack thereof) of oral hygiene were insufficient to sustain dental health. Once preventive care became a ritual, much of this chronic tooth decay was eradicated.

Likewise, at the turn of *this* century, the simple act of protecting and maintaining one's muscles and joints daily is not part of life's routine. In fact, when it comes to the health of the musculoskeletal system, the very notion of preventive care is nonexistent. This egregious neglect has led to tragic consequences. Chronic pain is a global epidemic, and the statistics are getting worse. By age 30, 7 of 10 people worldwide will have suffered some form of recurrent musculoskeletal pain; by age 50, almost everyone will experience a substantial, measurable loss in the functional capacity of their muscles and joints. The conventional wisdom is that that the human body is simply unable to last the span of a lifetime without the onset of dysfunction and pain. Nothing could be further from the truth. The fact is that the methods (or lack thereof) for taking care of one of the most fundamental aspects of the human body are insufficient to sustain its health. Once preventive musculoskeletal care becomes a ritual, nearly all of the aches and pain from which people suffer will be eradicated. But who knew? I certainly didn't.

I am pretty much your garden-variety American. My eating habits are spotty, I'm somewhat sedentary (although I do manage to exercise in spurts), I work excessively long hours, and, in spite of all that, am in excellent health. Nevertheless, I spent much of my adult life dodging bullets of pain. I experienced tension headaches and kinks in my neck as my stress levels rose, cramps in my hands and stiffness in my wrists from working on the computer, and aches in my knees and shin splints from my cardiovascular workouts. Sound familiar? I was also one of the millions of people who suffer from debilitating recurrent lower-back pain. To alleviate this plethora of chronic ailments, I went to chiropractors, acupuncturists, physicians, physiatrists, physical therapists, and massage therapists—all with no success. I bought a vast array of books on the subject, scoured the Internet for information, and paid oodles of money for inexplicably bizarre ergonomic contraptions. I even tried crystals! But all these attempts had the same results. It got to the point where I became resigned to suffering from chronic pain for the rest of my life. But when my pain went from being merely a nuisance to being absolutely debilitating, I lost all hope. It was in this state of desperation that I found my way to Dr. Weisberg's office. And that's when the quality of my life underwent a complete transformation. For it was during the initial visit that Dr. Weisberg introduced me to his revolutionary program.

The Weisberg Way is a three-tiered tactical strategy that facilitates optimal musculoskeletal health and longevity. It consists of the 3-Minute Maintenance Method for daily pain prevention, the Encyclopedia of Pain Relief for targeted rapid relief and reversal of preexisting conditions, and the 3-Month Tune-Up for maximizing the upkeep of the entire body. The first thing that appealed to me about the program was the small time commitment it required. I knew that I could realistically set aside three minutes a day to save myself weeks, months, even years of pain, no matter how busy my schedule. Then Dr. Weisberg explained to me the medical truths and science behind his unique philosophical outlook and methodological approach. Here was a commonsense, proactive, and self-managed program that within two days of its application produced a significant reduction in my symptoms! Within two weeks, I was completely pain free. I am thrilled to report that in the three years since fully incorporating this program into my life, I've had no recurrence of pain. Even more significantly, no *new* problems have developed.

In addition, all the members of my family are among the thousands of patients whom Dr. Weisberg has treated successfully. His methods have healed everyone, from my 9-year-old nephew to my 89-year-old grandmother. In fact, in my family alone, Dr. Weisberg has treated every body part from head to toe. By doing so, he has saved us all years of pain, unnecessary surgery, expensive doctor bills, and the prolonged intake of highly addictive medications. It occurred to me that since we benefited so greatly from the Weisberg Way, so could countless others; thus the inspiration for this book.

I am not a doctor or a nurse or associated with the medical profession in any way. I am a lay person who used to be in a lot of pain. That I no longer suffer is due solely to the Weisberg Way. Now I am able to work hard and play hard without life being hard as a result. The subtle addition to my morning routine—from brushing my teeth and having a cup of coffee to brushing my teeth, having a cup of coffee, *and* doing the 3-Minute Maintenance Method—has radically changed my life. Not only is there a vast qualitative difference today but I can finally look forward to a pain-free future. And you can too by making this simple program an essential part of your life.

Introduction
by Dr. Joseph Weisberg

I wrote this book to dramatically improve the quality of your life by teaching you how to go through it pain free. I wrote it to tell you that living pain free is not only possible but that right now, you possess all the tools you need to achieve that end. Armed with the information contained in these pages, you can *prevent* pain from occurring and *relieve* the pain you may already have. I will help you change the way you look at pain, change your understanding of human physiology, and change your ability to treat, heal, and keep yourself well. My program is designed to restore your body to optimal musculoskeletal health and maintain its inherent potential to stay there. I do this naturally: free of drugs, unproven herbal remedies, and expensive ergonomic equipment. Best of all, I do not ask that you alter your lifestyle or habits. All that is required of you is a little willingness and three minutes a day.

It's a little-known fact that the human body, barring disease or trauma (which falls outside the scope of this book), has the potential to function at a high level for more than a century. Maintained properly, your muscles and joints can last for 120 years. I know this sounds incomprehensible when most people do not make it to 60 years of age without pain, arthritis, stiffness, backaches, headaches, and general limited mobility. Even if you are not one of the hundreds of millions of people suffering from chronic pain, the statistics tell us that one day you most likely will be. We have become so conditioned to believe that pain is an inevitable part of aging that it is hard to believe that there is actually something that can be done about it. I'm here to tell you that there is.

More than 30 years ago I started developing my pain-prevention and rapid-relief program. Like so many inventions, mine was born out of necessity. Even as a highly trained and skilled physical therapist, I suffered from persistent and sometimes debilitating pain. After all, being a doctor did not make me immune to pain's onset. In fact, no one, irrespective of age, gender, or fitness level, is immune to its onset. When my pain became so severe that it interfered with my work and life, I knew I needed a solution to what had become an overwhelming problem. I looked for a program that would quickly relieve me of pain. Moreover, I wanted a way to stop the pain before it started. Alas, a program like that just did not exist. I searched my field and its companion literature, scoured bookstores and libraries, and even consulted other health professionals, to no avail. I kept getting the same advice, which may be familiar to you: take painkillers, continually seek profes-sional treatment, or have surgery. While these "remedies" sometimes temporarily relieved my pain, they did not cure it. As soon as the pain was gone, it seemed to immediately return. I knew there must be a better way.

I had an idea that was revolutionary then and remains so today: *Instead of treating the pain, I would treat the dysfunction that caused it in the first place.* You see, without even knowing it, you injure yourself in countless little ways every day. Com-mon activities, such as reaching for a bag of groceries, lifting your briefcase, running for a train, walking the dog, sitting at your desk, working at the computer, brushing your hair, exercising, and thousands of others, can subtly traumatize your muscles and joints. When you string enough of these little injuries, or microtraumas, to-gether, the result is pain. However, I knew from my work that muscles and joints have a remarkable built-in capacity to bounce back from the use and abuse they are subjected to. I designed my program to harness the body's natural restorative powers daily, thereby preventing these little injuries from accumulating and doing harm. As I began to explore why musculoskeletal anatomy is so susceptible to wear and tear, I found that there is a wide gap between this system's biological needs and the modern lifestyle. Because my program supplements this deficiency, it is the missing link. I will explain all of this to you in detail throughout the book, but for now, suffice it to say that I developed a program of therapeutic movements that *enables the body to protect itself from itself.* I call this program the Weisberg Way.

I had one final criterion that would complete my program: economizing time. I have always been an active and busy man, too busy, in fact, to allocate a portion of the day to the upkeep of my physical well-being. For someone in my profession, you would think this would not be so. However, spare time is something I've never had much of, even to spend on a program that would empower my life and save me pain, frustration, and money. Knowing that I am not unique in this respect, I wanted to make the Weisberg Way fit into one's life rather than having to fit one's life around it. I was keenly aware that a program must be practical for it to be done consistently and, therefore, effectively. As I researched the medical literature I discovered that, indeed, less is more: Three minutes a day is not just sufficient, it is more than enough to maintain optimal musculoskeletal health. My program was now complete.

The first patient to test the Weisberg Way was a natural choice: me! After I confirmed its safety and effectiveness, I began imparting the program to my patients. The early Weisberg Way Warriors, as I have come to call them, reported what I had already experienced. After just a few weeks, they became *more* active with *less* pain. As time went on, their pain vanished completely. As I followed up after a year, two years, even a decade, I found that those patients who adhered to the Weisberg Way had little likelihood of recurrence. Since then, I have helped thousands of patients achieve the same results. Now I am passing my methods on to you.

3 Minutes to a Pain-Free Life is the key to releasing you from the seemingly inescapable prison of pain. This book will make it possible for you to walk through the door leading to a life of greater health and vitality. By reading this introduction, you have already taken the first step on your journey toward a pain-free life.

Part I

The Problem Is Not the Problem

1: The Good News About Pain

I HAVE A LITTLE ANECDOTE I like to tell my patients when they first come to see me: I've got some good news and some bad news for you. First the bad news: You're in pain. Now the good news: You're in pain.

Sounds ridiculous? It does to my patients as well, that is until I give them the same information I'm about to give you. By the time you're done reading this chapter, you will begin to look at pain differently and see it for what it really is: a teacher guiding you to a complete and accurate accounting of what problems are occurring in your body.

All pain serves a purpose. You have to understand the protective language of your body so that you can respond to it appropriately.

Pain is not your enemy. In fact, it is one of your greatest allies. The simple truth is that pain is nature's perfect alarm system, designed to alert you that something is wrong. When this alarm goes off, you are being sent an unmistakable message that something happening inside or to your body is causing you harm. Why is it so imperative for you to see pain in this light? Because misconstruing or ignoring what your body is trying to tell you can have grave, even crippling, consequences. I am going to teach you how to recognize and interpret the signals of pain so that you may heed the sirens of this built-in warning system.

I know it may be hard to perceive pain as anything but bad, especially when you or someone you know is suffering. And a whole lot of people are suffering. Pain does not discriminate. It can strike whether you are a young adult or of advanced age, male or female, rich or poor. It doesn't matter if you are a high-performance athlete or a couch potato, a yogi or a mommy. I am well aware from my own experiences how much being in pain reduces your zest for living. It robs you of the ability to be up for all the challenges and good times that life has to offer and seems to hurt much more than it can ever possibly help. And to a certain extent that's true, especially if you're talking about the kind of pain that just won't go away. However, I am not suggesting that I think it's a good thing to *stay* in pain. In fact, I wrote this book so that you could live your life pain free. I want to help you develop a deeper relationship and connection with your body than you've ever had before. When you make a friend of pain, you will be acknowledging and respecting the intricacies and nuances of your body's design. Thus the first step toward living a pain-free life is understanding that *the good news about pain is that you can feel it.*

Without the ability to feel pain, you would be unable to survive. (Until recently, children who were born lacking this faculty had an extremely diminished life expectancy.)[1] It is one of creation's great paradoxes that you incur pain in order to avert pain. Think about it. Pain makes it possible to navigate your way through the perils that are often a part of daily life. For instance, when you touch a hot stove, the pain you feel demands that you pull your hand away to avoid any additional harm. If you suffer an injury, such as a fractured leg, the pain prohibits any further use of the limb until it has healed. Likewise, if you develop a disease or suffer a major trauma, the body responds by sending a clear directive to your brain: Pay attention and take action now.

Not all pain is created equal. Although it may feel the same, there are actually different kinds of pain. They are generally broken down into two categories: acute pain (sharp, intense, immediate) and chronic pain (recurrent, persistent, long-lasting). In the preceding paragraph, all of the examples illustrated acute pain. This type of pain is characterized as an instantaneous symptom of a specific injury triggered by some form of tissue damage. Acute pain can be mild, such as

A Journey Down Pain's Pathway

Your ability to say "ouch!" is preceded by a complex series of electrochemical impulses triggered when your body suffers an unpleasant or harmful stimulus. You don't really "feel" pain until your *brain* receives these impulses, sent from the injured tissue by *peripheral nerves* through your *spinal cord*, and interprets them as messages of warning. Your peripheral nerves are a network of fibers that branch throughout your body. At the end of some of these fibers are *nociceptors*, whose function is to sense tissue damage and other danger. Millions of nociceptors in your skin, joints, muscles, bones, and around your internal organs send electrical impulses along the peripheral nerves. When these impulses reach your spinal cord, they are filtered and sorted. Severe injuries are given high priority and sent on instantaneously; less severe injuries take a little longer to reach their destination, the brain. Once they are there, a series of involuntary and voluntary actions are initiated to rectify the situation that caused the pain.

from a splinter, or it can be severe, such as when you have a tooth pulled. Its duration can vary from a matter of seconds, such as from a stubbed toe, or to several months, such as from a bad burn. The important distinguishing factor is that there is a direct correlation between cause (injury) and effect (pain). In addition, there is a reasonable, almost predictable amount of time between effect (pain) and recovery (no pain). Treating acute pain is also fairly predictable because the injury itself informs you of what needs to be done to remedy the problem. Whether you can manage this treatment yourself, such as by putting a Band-Aid on a minor cut, or require medical assistance, such as needing stitches for a severe cut, there are some obvious steps that will eventually lead to the alleviation of your pain. In other words, when you fix what's wrong, the pain goes away. All of these factors make it easy to see why feeling acute pain is so vital to our existence. However, things become a lot less clear when we start talking about the main focus of this book: chronic musculoskeletal pain.

Chronic Pain: The Inside Story

No two words put together back to back inspire more fear, spark as much controversy, and cause as much confusion as "chronic pain." You cannot turn on the television, listen to the radio, open a newspaper, or surf the Internet without being bombarded by a plethora of information on this subject. I have found a lot of this information unnecessarily complex, often conflicting, and sometimes even highly inaccurate. Everyone, it seems, is talking about chronic pain because everyone, it seems, is in it. And that's no exaggeration. It has, quite literally, become an epidemic. The statistics in the United States alone are staggering:

- More than 100 million people suffer from chronic pain.[2]

- 90 percent of the population will experience back pain during their lives.[3]

- 70 million workdays are lost from pain a year, costing industry more than $100 billion a year in lost wages and insurance.[4]

- 50 million people are partially or totally disabled by their chronic or long-term pain.[5]

- 45 million people have severe and chronic headaches.[6]

- 40 million people suffer from arthritis, 26 million of them women.[7]

- 20 million people experience jaw and lower-facial pain.[8]

- 10 million children under the age of 18 suffer from chronic pain.[9]

- 6 million people suffer from fibromyalgia, a general diagnosis for the myriad aches and pains afflicting muscles, joints, and tendons.[10]

You may be reading this book because you are already one of these statistics. Or you may be reading it because you don't want to become one of them. Either way, the information in this book will provide you with the help you're looking for. I'm going to let you in on a little secret: *In nearly 100 percent of these cases of chronic musculoskeletal pain, the symptoms can be rapidly relieved and the conditions themselves prevented.*

The word "chronic" comes from the Greek word for "time." Generally speaking, chronic pain could be characterized as any pain that recurs or persists over an indeterminate period of time. Like acute pain, chronic pain can run the gamut from mild to severe; and the duration of each bout can last from minutes to months, even years. What distinguishes the two is that while the source of acute pain can be attributed to an obvious injury or illness, many who suffer from chronic pain (barring the chronic pain associated with disease, such as cancer, or trauma, such as the chronic pain associated with nerve damage) do so seemingly in the *absence* of an injury. For instance, how many times have you experienced pain that seemed to just pop up out of nowhere? How many times have you said that "without warning" you couldn't move your neck or that "suddenly" your back went out? If these experiences are true for you, you're not alone. Millions of people around the world have reported the same thing. Likewise, whereas the recovery from acute pain seems to follow logically from the treatment of the injury itself, chronic pain persists in spite of, sometimes even because of, treatment. In fact, quite often there seems to be no logic at all; no discernible direct link between cause, effect, and temporary recovery. Chronic pain seems to come as mysteriously as it goes. Of course, there is a reason for the sudden onset and dissipation of chronic pain, as I am about to show you, but the lack of objective evidence pinpointing an actual injury has led to a great debate in the medical community on the very nature of chronic pain.

Because of its vexing and ambiguous qualities, many health professionals have been reluctant to even acknowledge chronic pain as a real ailment. I cannot tell you how many patients have come to me over the years after their doctors told them that their pain was imaginary, a manifestation of hypochondria, or a desperate ploy for attention. Although I am always appalled when I hear this, I am never surprised. Western medicine is dependent upon the tangible for analysis and care—seeing, cutting, poking, and prodding. But chronic pain is intangible and cannot be quantified by most extrinsic standards, except that the patient is clearly feeling something. Because many of the empirical methods commonly used today for diagnosing chronic pain, such as CAT scans, MRIs, X-rays, and blood tests, are inadequate for formulating proper treatment, many doctors feel frustrated and impotent in the face of the growing crisis. Some have even dismissed it altogether. The situation has become as critical as it has in large part from widespread misdiagnosis, mistreatment, and ignorance.

The failure on the part of many health professionals to adequately deal with chronic pain exacts a devastating psychological toll on its sufferers. To be in physical pain is bad enough; to be given little support and offered no solution only leaves one feeling utterly helpless and depressed. The severity of this emotional trauma cannot be overestimated. Fifty percent of suicides give pain as motivation.[11] Changing the approach to chronic pain has literally become a matter of life or death. Lately, the medical community has acknowledged an urgent need to reassess their position, and slowly a new attitude and understanding is emerging. Not long ago I was reading an article in *Newsweek* that stated:

> Realizing that for years doctors neglected to include pain management
>
> in patient care, the medical establishment has, over the past decade,
>
> taken a new, more aggressive approach to treating pain. . . . Even
>
> Congress has gotten into the act [by] passing a law declaring the next
>
> 10 years the "Decade of Pain Control and Research."[12]

Of course, chronic pain is real. But even coming up with a singular and coherent definition has proved difficult. It's not that there isn't one; in fact, there are too many. It reminds me of the old joke: "What do you get when you ask three doctors a question? Five answers and a second opinion." Most health professionals agree that chronic pain is pain that reappears over and over. I can tell you that defining it that way is simply not enough. While it may be accurate, it does not sufficiently convey a complete picture of the condition. Why? Mainly because of what it leaves out. For instance, what causes pain to reappear? What causes it to disappear? Is there a cause in the first place? There is, of course, a more precise definition. After spending more than 30 years in clinical practice, research, and teaching, my definition is this: *Chronic pain (outside the realm of disease or trauma) is recurrent and persistent pain related to the biomechanical dysfunction of muscles and joints.* Understanding *why* this is so, from a physiological point of view, will be explored more fully in Chapter 3, although I will touch upon it here. The important concept of this chapter is *what* this pain is telling you, and *how* this information can be correctly applied toward maintaining and maximizing your all-around health.

Conditions That Cause Chronic Pain

Chronic pain, like acute pain, is a warning sign that something is wrong. Whereas acute pain is indicative of an overt problem, chronic pain is indicative of an underlying one. More specifically, it is an indication that the mechanical function of your musculoskeletal system has been compromised in some way. When you have a headache or a backache, when your hip hurts or your neck is tight, you are being sent a clear message that the muscles and joints in that area are, to varying degrees of severity, impaired. Chronic pain is, therefore, a direct result of injury. Whereas acute pain is the result of a singular, often perceptible injury in which the tissue is *damaged,* chronic pain is the result of multiple imperceptible injuries in which the tissue is *irritated.* In some instances chronic pain can trace its source to an illness or a catastrophic event, but it mostly occurs as a consequence of an infinite series of benign actions that subtly harm the muscles and joints. When does this happen? Every time we move.

The human body was designed for motion, and motion is made possible by a complex interplay between our muscles and joints. We need to move in order to sustain ourselves, whether to procure food and shelter, to get from here to there, or simply to avoid the atrophy that is guaranteed to set in with inertia. Yet movement itself can be harmful to the very anatomy that makes it feasible in the first place. Flawless as the design of the musculoskeletal system is, it is prone to wear and tear as it endures the constant rigors of use, misuse, and abuse. You may be thinking that this wear and tear must be caused only by severe or radical activity, but I can tell you that it's not. Common and *unavoidable* activities that make up daily life, such as sitting, walking, standing, reaching, grabbing, and holding, are some of the main culprits. Although the degree to which the musculoskeletal system is vulnerable to wear and tear correlates directly to how well its functional health is maintained, these seemingly innocuous actions are likely to produce injuries, which are called *microtraumas,* or small wounds (in contrast to acute pain, which is caused by *macrotraumas,* or large wounds). Taken by themselves, these microtraumas have very little effect on the structure and function of the body. In fact, they are so tiny that they occur silently and evade detection. Slipping under the radar, they fail to trigger the healing process, which begins only when the body senses a direct or immediate threat (as it does with an acute macrotrauma). Overlooked and untreated by the body itself, these microtraumas accumulate, resulting in the deterioration of the tissues of the muscles and joints. This minute deterioration is responsible for the most caustic and debilitating chronic pain.

Chronic musculoskeletal pain is like an echo. The pain you feel in the present is the delayed effect of the seeds of biomechanical dysfunction that were sown in the past. In other words, chronic pain is the end result of the abnormal performance of the anatomy responsible for movement. As the dysfunction grows, which it surely will if microtraumas are allowed to amass unchecked, the functional capacity of your musculoskeletal system continues to diminish. Because your muscles and joints try to compensate for the dysfunction by adapting to the abnormalities, the entire structure is subject to overload and stress. Encumbered by the excessive burden muscles impose on the joints, thus inhibiting the full range of motion required for their

Biomechanical dysfunction is . . .

- **Tight, stiff, or short muscles**
- **Weak and imbalanced musculature**
- **Lack of lubrication in the joints**
- **Misalignment of the joints**
- **Poor posture**

lubrication and nourishment. This situation is so precarious that little provocation is needed to upset the delicate balance of the system. Thus even the slightest movement can cause the sudden onset of a great deal of pain. That is how your lower back goes out from your just bending down. Or how your neck becomes immobile after you barely turn your head sideways. Or how you are stricken by blinding pain in your arm after simply lifting your cell phone. In reality, there is noth-ing sudden about the onset at all. Chronic pain is a manifestation of the gradual buildup of a festering dysfunction that has remained dormant until now.

The funny thing about your muscles and joints is that although they are prone to injury, they are also incredibly resilient and have a remarkable ability to bounce back from the daily grind. The musculoskeletal system is capable of re-pairing itself, and it strives to return itself to a state of health. Left to its own de-vices, it will attempt to restore function to a degree of normalcy, and in some ways it does so successfully. This explains how bouts of chronic pain seem to suddenly dissipate. As the system adjusts to the buildup of microtraumas, the symptoms (pain) subside. However, there is real danger in thinking that the absence of pain means the absence of dysfunction. The relief, as it often turns out, is temporary, because the underlying problem, which is the constant wear and tear to your mus-cles and joints, has not been solved. This in turn leaves the door wide open for even the simplest of tasks to induce another episode. Thus the vicious cycle of chronic pain plays itself out.

You may be wondering if this cycle can ever be broken or if it is possible to successfully navigate a course through life free of pain when we are in an almost constant state of motion and even ordinary activities can be injurious. The answer to these questions is unequivocally Yes! There is a way to properly prepare your mus-culoskeletal system for everyday use, safeguard against the inevitable wear and tear, and nurture its innate ability to remain healthy. And that way is the Weisberg Way.

The Weisberg Way

The foundation of my program is the principle that one of the most potent and ef-fective tools for healing the body is the body itself. Although movement can dam-age the muscles and joints when there is an underlying dysfunction, *properly designed movement* can affect its recovery. The Weisberg Way takes the body through six different 30-second therapeutic movements (TMs) that combat chronic pain by eliminating the cause of its occurrence. How? By healing microtraumatic effects, thus preventing their harmful accumulation: by taking joints through their full range of motion, guaranteeing their full lubrication: and by keeping the major muscle groups at their proper length, ensuring that they are ready for any activity you choose. And the Weisberg Way doesn't require a lot of time or effort. In fact, a little goes a long way when it comes to keeping your muscles and joints in optimal health. Three minutes, to be exact.

The Weisberg Way techniques include:

- The 3-Minute Maintenance Method: my daily program, made up of six 30-second therapeutic movements (TMs), which improves and maintains your optimal musculoskeletal health while preventing nearly all types of general aches and pains.

- The Encyclopedia of Pain Relief: a series of targeted, body-part-specific TMs that rapidly relieve existing pain from head to toe.

- The 3-Month Tune-Up: a series of diagnostic tests and TMs applied once every three months that tune up and monitor the health of your body.

Treated to a daily and consistent application of my program, your musculoskeletal system can remain in excellent condition for more than a hundred years! Without it, whether you are now in pain or not, your muscles and joints will eventually fall prey to irreversible erosion and damage. It is important to understand that the simple act of living is the basis and foundation for the conditions that lead to chronic pain. We are all at risk. No one is exempt. While most people do not feel the full-blown effects of dysfunction until later in life, one way or another, either through recurrent episodic flare-ups or the inability to move the way you used to, the cumulative buildup will catch up with you. Yet I have met very few people who think about the upkeep of their musculoskeletal system. Of the rare individuals who do bother to think about it, I haven't met a single one who knows how to do so, or, more accurately, how to properly do so.

For those of you that think that going to the gym or taking an aerobics class is the same thing as tending to the biological needs of your muscles and joints, think again. Exercises that target strength, aesthetics, and even agility, while important, do not result in biomechanical health. We are prompted to watch our diets and eat right. We are encouraged to get in shape and exercise consistently. We diligently go for regular checkups and take care of our teeth, our eyes, and our hearts and other internal organs. We are even conscious of the role that our external environment plays in our well-being. And yet neglect runs rampant when it comes to taking care of our muscles and joints. Although they account for more than 60 percent of the makeup of our bodies and their health determines the very quality of our lives, their preservation is taken for granted. What good, I often wonder, is the pursuit of all-around health when we—children, adults, and senior citizens alike—cannot move without it hurting? What good is an increasing life expectancy when those extra years are mired in disability, immobility, and suffering? It requires so little to achieve so much, yet musculoskeletal health is not a priority. Honestly, when was the last time you thought about allocating a portion of your day to the preservation of your muscles and joints? I'm sure that before reading this book, you probably didn't even know that you could or should.

Now you know better. You know that you can engage yourself in a program that will keep your musculoskeletal system in optimal health for the rest of your life. That's why I wrote this book. I want *you* to have the power to manage your musculoskeletal treatment and care. Should symptoms arise, which they may as a result of the condition of your muscles and joints or your lifestyle and habits, you will have the ability not only to stop the symptoms but also any progression. Furthermore, you can *reverse* many of the conditions you may already have, such as some forms of arthritis, and return your body to normal function. Some of my chief goals are to make you independent of running to the doctor, incurring invasive surgery, investing in expensive ergonomic equipment, and taking highly addictive drugs or unproven herbal remedies in an effort to make and keep yourself well. I can tell you that these choices are frequently unnecessary, ineffective, and sometimes responsible for making the situation worse. You will find that employing the Weisberg Way will provide you with all the help you need. To as-

If your musculoskeletal health is diminished, don't worry. You have the power to restore it.

sess what course of action is the most appropriate to take for your musculoskeletal care, I will supply you with all the information necessary to make prudent and informed decisions rather than uneducated or desperate ones. To that end, I have developed six basic tenets that you should make the cornerstone of your new approach to pain relief and prevention.

Prescription for Relief and Prevention

1. Don't Put the Pain Alarm on Snooze

It will go off again. And I can assure you that when it does, the pain will have been made worse by the wear. Yet the second that alarm sounds, most of us want to shut it down immediately by whatever means possible. Desperate to alleviate the pain, we reach out for one of the abundant over-the-counter or prescription drugs available today. In the year 2000 alone, Americans spent more than $4 billion on anti-inflammatories[13] and close to $2 billion on narcotics.[14] (Abuse of the latter is fast becoming an epidemic unto itself. I will discuss more of the pros and cons of pain medications in Chapter 4.) Ironically, many of these medications can actually inhibit the healing process. Thus they increase rather than reduce the amount of time you're in pain. Furthermore, by masking pain, these treatments enable you to continue doing the activities that produced the problem in the first place. This perpetuates an endless continuum of injury begetting injury. Making the *pain* go away will not make the *problem* go away. In fact, the opposite is usually true. Temporary relief can cause permanent problems. I am interested in providing you with permanent relief, which renders your problems temporary.

Here's my golden rule of pain: *If you can feel it, you can deal with it. If you can't, you won't.* Think of it this way: Would you have an elaborate fire alarm system installed in your home only to disable it because the sound of the alarm is annoying? If you do disable it, the only way you'll be able to tell if there's a fire is when the whole house is already engulfed in flames. Doesn't make sense, right? Of course not. So why treat your body that way? Instead, let the pain sirens blare so that you can tend to the danger before it's too late.

2. Listen to Your Body

Your body has a lot of vital information to tell you, and, as we saw earlier, the only way it can communicate it to your brain is by the nerves. When something goes wrong, your body alerts you to this danger by sending a messenger—pain—to deliver its message of warning. It hurts so that it can help. I have spent this entire chapter trying to impress upon you one point: You need to pay close attention to these signs, no matter how minor or major your discomfort may be. Pain is a sign that harm has befallen you, and it is sending you a clear directive that your immediate care is required.

Remarkably, most people don't bother to listen. They deal with their pain by not dealing with it at all. Instead, they choose to simply ignore it. Because chronic pain is caused by a gradual buildup of dysfunction, there are usually many warning signs that occur before a full-blown episode. Yet many patients come to me when their pain is so bad that they are completely unable to function. When I ask them why they waited so long before they sought help, they respond, "I was hoping that it would just go away." It won't. The first step toward any solution is acknowledging the problem. When it comes to eradicating pain, you must start by listening.

3. Know Your ABCs

You had to study your ABCs when you were learning to read and write. In essence, you are learning a new language now: the language of pain. Once you start listening to your body, you will notice that pain manifests itself in a variety of ways. Different types of pain indicate different types of problems. Because there is a tendency to lump all pain together, these subtle distinctions are often missed. It is not enough to just listen to pain; you need to be able to distinguish among its attributes to understand what it is trying to tell you. Specifically, is it symptomatic of a pathology that may need further investigation, or is it symptomatic of a chronic musculoskeletal condition that you can correct on your own with the Weisberg Way? Making this determination is crucial because it will indicate how you should proceed. This step and the ones that follow are designed to help you properly evaluate your symptoms so that you may make a correct self-diagnosis.

When you are suffering from a chronic musculoskeletal condition, the pain will usually express itself in one or more of the following three ways: Aching, Burning, and Cramping.

ACHING Aching, by far the most common of the three, is a dull, continuous pain that is usually mild to moderate in nature. Although its onset is slow, it gradually worsens with time. A single episode can span a day, as with a recurrent, nagging headache, or it can span the course of weeks, months, even years, as with a backache. Aching usually is an indication that the muscles and joints have been subjected to the buildup of microtraumas in that area. As microtraumas continue to evolve unabated, this mechanical irritation causes the muscles to contract and tighten and the joints to erode. When this happens, they irritate the adjacent nerves, which in turn causes the area to emit an aching sensation.

Aching can also be caused by a chemical irritation to the nerves. For instance, when you overwork your muscles, say, from lifting weights or handling something heavy, they are unable to dispose of the excess metabolic waste material produced during this strenuous activity. This extraneous waste irritates the nerve endings, which cause the aching condition known as a charley horse.

Aching from mechanical or chemical irritations is an indicator of underlying musculoskeletal dysfunction and is treated by correcting that dysfunction.

BURNING Burning is characterized by its fast, abrupt onset and is considerably more severe and pronounced than a general ache. It too is the result of an underlying dysfunction from the buildup of microtraumas that, in this case, causes a reduction of circulation to the area. When muscles are deprived of blood flow, they cannot properly flush away the normal metabolic waste that is produced during all movement. Burning is the by-product of this deprivation.

Burning usually occurs when you exert yourself and push your body to its physical limit. Whereas aching can arise from even the simplest activity (or none at all), burning usually comes about when you engage your muscles in activities that go beyond what they are accustomed to or prepared for. Once you stop engaging the muscle in the activity, the burning usually subsides.

CRAMPING Cramping is a sudden and intensely painful contraction of a muscle. This spasmodic sensation is immediate and extremely sharp, but it usually doesn't last or linger for long. It's not hard to recognize when you have a cramp: The pain is so great that it renders the area immobile. The most frequent cause is from some form of physical overexertion, such as participation in exercise for which your muscles and joints are unprepared. It can also arise from putting your muscles into positions to which they are ill-equipped, such as repeatedly wearing tightly fitting or high-heeled shoes. In fact, the most common areas of affliction are the legs and feet.

When a short, weak, or overused muscle becomes fatigued, it is deprived of nutrients and oxygen, which causes a buildup of lactic acid to occur. When this buildup becomes too great, the muscle reacts by cramping. Of the three, cramping is the hardest to ignore (which you now know you should never do with any pain), yet the easiest to treat. Either a stretch or massage will generally alleviate it.

If your pain falls into one of these categories, there is a high likelihood that what you feel is symptomatic of chronic musculoskeletal pain. And that's the really good news, because, as you may have noticed, almost all of these symptoms are caused by physical or, more specifically, biomechanical limitations that can be permanently corrected with the Weisberg Way. Yes, it can be tricky trying to pinpoint which of the ABCs you are feeling at a given moment. It is possible to erroneously classify aching as burning, cramping as aching, and so on. However, distinguishing from among the three isn't really necessary, for all are indicative of the same thing. It is important, however, for you to be able to characterize your pain as falling somewhere within these categories, regardless of how vague or definitive this characterization may be. Knowing your ABCs will make it possible for you to interpret your pain thoroughly and accurately.

If aching, burning, or cramping doesn't seem to properly describe or convey the essence of pain you're feeling, it doesn't mean that your symptoms don't fall within these categories. The ABCs are comprehensive, not exhaustive. There may be a word or words that is more suitable than aching, burning, or cramping. Chances are, though, that these words are synonymous with one of the ABCs. For instance, "throbbing," "pounding," "gnawing," "stabbing," "pulling," and "tender" are all common words used to describe chronic musculoskeletal pain. (In contrast, "shooting," "paralyzing," "dizzying," "nauseating," and "blinding" are words often used to describe pain that is symptomatic of trauma and disease.) There are many ways people articulate their pain, and it is impossible for me to include them all, especially the ones that aren't real words. (I once had a patient who told me that her pain was "stingulizing" her. Perplexed, I asked what she meant by that. She said that her arm was stinging and immobilized; thus stingulizing. After examining her, I concluded that she meant a burning sensation caused by continuous overexertion of the area.) Furthermore, sometimes it's hard to determine, even for yourself, what exactly it is that you are feeling. Pain is both subjective and objective at the same time. Thus your subjective interpretation of your own pain may in fact differ substantially from the objective truth of what that pain really is. So something that feels like a burn to you may in fact be an ache. Although classification may be challenging, it is your job to try to characterize what you're feeling in some way to see if it fits in or correlates somehow to the ABCs.

If your pain falls outside of the ABCs, that doesn't automatically mean that you are suffering from another form of pathology, not from a chronic musculoskeletal condition. Likewise, just because your pain falls into one of these categories doesn't mean that it is a chronic musculoskeletal condition, not another form of pathology. There are some additional criteria that need to be met to positively identify chronic musculoskeletal pain from among the myriad other possible ailments. This brings us to our next step.

4. Think About Action and Position

Chronic musculoskeletal pain is caused by something you did to or with your body. This is what distinguishes it from pathology or disease, which often occurs without relevance to or in spite of what may you may or may not have done with your body. It follows that one of the most important criteria in establishing whether you have a musculoskeletal condition is your ability to connect it with its cause. Earlier in the chapter I explained how everyday movements are responsible for most chronic pain. To make the link between cause and effect, you need to understand the two elements that make up movement: action and position.

ACTION Action is the way you use your body. Specifically, it refers to the infinite variety of activities you engage in. This includes walking, running, stepping, dancing, lifting, throwing, raising your arms, reaching out, and turning your neck. While each instance of an action does not necessarily cause pain, its repetition can. Why? When your body is not in optimal musculoskeletal condition, every time you repeat a certain activity, the microtraumas produced by that activity accumulate. It's a bit like a train wreck in that they keep piling up, one on top of the other. Eventually, if left untreated, the accumulation will escalate to higher levels. As that happens, you feel pain. It is your job to evaluate which actions may have caused your current condition. That's not as hard as you might think. To illustrate, let me cite you the example of my coauthor.

Ms. Shink first contacted me when she had excruciating lower-back pain. Because she lives on one coast and I on the other, we had to establish by phone whether her pain was musculoskeletal in nature. So I went looking for a cause. I began by asking her what kinds of activities she participates in. She told me that though she usually jogs and lifts weights, she hadn't for some time because she was busy writing a new book. A very interesting clue, I thought. Then I asked her what she was doing when her pain appeared. She told me that she was just sitting at her computer, almost completely stationary. This was, in fact, the way she had spent her days for many months. Another clue. That alone could have been the culprit, but I decided to probe a little deeper. And this is where the mystery unraveled. She went on to tell me that while sitting at her computer she had to constantly twist her body and bend down because her pencil sharpener was on a shelf below her desk. Ten, twenty times a day, week after week, she bent over in this fashion with no problem. Eventually, though, this repetitive activity caused a chain reaction to occur, whereby one more time became the "one time too many." By thinking about action, we were able to clearly identify and establish the precise cause of her pain.

POSITION Position is the passive placement of your muscles and joints before and during an action. Specifically, it refers to the length of the muscle and the angle of the joint from the start through the end of an action. Often it is the way we position our bodies, not the activity itself, that causes us the most pain. In other words, it's not what you're doing, but how you're doing it that counts. When you engage your body in an action, whether static or fluid, your muscles and joints adjust to accommodate themselves to it. Sustaining the action requires an enormous expenditure of energy on their part. Eventually, if you fix yourself in a position, such as sitting or in a poor posture, for an extended period of time, the muscles will shorten or elongate their length in an effort to conserve energy. Elongated muscles lose their strength, and shortened muscles are tight and less flexible. Both put stress on the joints, which makes the entire structure highly prone to injury. In addition, changing your position forces the muscles to go outside the range of their newly formed lengths. This strain causes pain. In the previous example of Ms. Shink, her pain could just as easily have been attributed to sitting at the computer for 8 to 10 hours a day. Why? Because when she was hunched over and fixed like that, some of her muscles assumed a very short position. Just standing up could have triggered a great deal of pain. In my estimation, it was the combination of action and position—bending down and sitting for long periods of time—that induced her episode.

To establish the link between the position of your muscles and joints, and your pain, look at the way you handle your body. Do you keep it in one position for long periods, causing the muscles to shorten? Do you participate in activities, such as ballet dancing or yoga, that cause the muscles to elongate? Thinking about position will often help you identify the culprit, even when it seems that there is none.

The goal in establishing this link is to determine whether the pain you are feeling is musculoskeletal in nature. If you have concluded that your pain is not, you should seek advice from a health care professional. If you have concluded that it is, you can use the Weisberg Way to relieve this pain. An added bonus is that my program also prepares your muscles and joints for the continuation of the activity you have isolated as the cause of your pain. I want to make it very clear that *you do not need to stop doing this activity; rather that you need to prepare your body for it.* I want you to have the freedom to play now without having to pay later. When you take care of your muscles and joints, they will take care of you.

5. Make a Self-Diagnosis

You *do* have the ability to make a self-diagnosis. After you've completed steps 1 through 4, it's time to take the following evaluative tests to ensure that your analysis is complete. (If, after completing these tests, the exact nature of your pain remains unclear, you should consult a trusted health care professional to help you reach a more accurate conclusion.)

First, the Chronic Musculoskeletal Pain Test is a quick checklist that you can refer to any time you're in pain.

Chronic Musculoskeletal Pain Test

☐ 1. Can your pain be described as one or more of the ABCs (Aching, Burning, Cramping)?

☐ 2. Is your pain associated with action and position?

☐ 3. Was the onset of your pain gradual?

☐ 4. Have you ever felt pain in this area before?

☐ 5. When you move the painful area, do you hear body noise, like clicking or grinding?

☐ 6. If you try to give the area resistance, like pushing against it or forcing the muscle to contract, does the pain increase?

☐ 7. Is your range of motion in the area limited in any way?

If you answered Yes to one or more of these questions, it is highly likely that the pain you feel is musculoskeletal in nature and that its treatment is manageable through one or more of the Weisberg Way techniques. Please note: The more questions you answered Yes to, the more certain your self-diagnosis is.

Second, the Nonchronic Musculoskeletal Pain Test is an important diagnostic tool to ensure that you're not suffering from a disease that affects your muscles and joints.

Nonchronic Musculoskeletal Pain Test

☐ 1. **Does the description of your pain fall outside the scope of the ABCs (Aching, Burning, Cramping)?**

☐ 2. **Did your pain suddenly appear with no relationship to action or position?**

☐ 3. **In the absence of a traumatic event, injury, or previous history of pain in this area, is it very severe?**

☐ 4. **Is your pain steady and continuous?**

☐ 5. **Did your pain ever awaken you in the middle of the night?**

☐ 6. **Does it take more effort now to do simple tasks, even in the absence of pain?**

☐ 7. **Is the pain itself causing a systemic reaction, such as vomiting or diarrhea?**

If you answered Yes to one or more of these questions, you should contact a health professional and further investigate the source of your pain, as it may be indicative of a condition that falls outside the scope of this book.

6. Live in the Solution

The alternative to living in the solution is to live with the problem, which means the continuation and progression of your pain. It also means the cumulative deterioration of your muscles and joints, which ensures that your next episode of chronic pain will be worse than your last one. If you're sick and tired of being sick and tired, you are sufficiently motivated to make some fundamental changes in your life. I know that's a hard thing to do, even if you're aware of how the quality of your life will vastly improve if you make them. It seems that part of human nature is to become comfortable with being uncomfortable. But I am convinced that given the right tools and information, you can affect healthy change. That's why I made the Weisberg Way as practical as I could without sacrificing its ability to remain effective. I want the incorporation of my program into your life to be as easy on you as possible, so that you can become and remain well. Three minutes a day is all it takes to transform the way you feel, the way you age, what you're able to do and how you do it, and whether you will spend your life in moderate to debilitating pain or pain free.

Living in the solution means choosing to make the Weisberg Way one of your daily rituals. It means employing the strategies that I have laid out for you in this chapter at the first sign of pain and using the information contained in the rest of this book as a vital resource and companion guide in your effort to achieve optimal musculoskeletal health. It means setting these goals and being okay with the possibility that you may not always accomplish them perfectly. And it means tuning into the positive messages of pain and tuning out the negative ones. Living in the solution is transforming your body from a painful liability to a pain-free asset.

Happy Endings: Stella's Story

Stella F. is a 90-year-old woman with two children, seven grandchildren, and five great-grandchildren. She led a very active life until her mid-70s, when she began experiencing severe, debilitating pain in her lower back and legs. For many years, Stella suffered from the symptoms of stenosis (the narrowing of the canals in the lumbar region of the spine) and from osteoarthritis of the knees. She came to see me shortly after her orthopedist diagnosed her condition as "beyond repair." By that time, nearly a decade ago, she was almost completely immobile.

In 1993 my doctor told me that I would never walk again. This was a terrible shock. I always prided myself on being able to keep up with my large family, even the younger members. In fact, I had spent much of my life running around, going from place to place, involved in all sorts of adventures. But when I turned 80 (a youngster!), I couldn't even make my way across a room. With no solutions available—surgery and medicines were deemed too risky at my age—I was wheelchair-bound. While this was very disheartening, I honestly thought that it was just a natural part of life. After all, the vast majority of the people I knew of similar age were going through exactly the same thing as me. Our bodies were falling apart. It seemed that the golden years weren't filled with very much gold. That is, until I went to Dr. Weisberg.

Dr. Weisberg got me walking again. How was he able to do what no other doctor or health professional could? The first step on my road to recovery was regaining my hope. Dr. Weisberg assured me that neither my age nor the arthritic changes in my back and knees would hinder my ability to be well again. He showed me countless studies and told me of many of his elderly patients who had restored pain-free function and health to their muscles and joints. And these were cases that were as bad, if not worse, than my own.

Then he taught me how to make good use of my pain. Instead of searching for ways to stop feeling it, I started using pain as a guide. I began to realize that pain let me know which activities were safe to embrace and which I should avoid. This was a big turning point because I was no longer afraid that moving would hurt me. As my confidence with my pain alarm system grew, I slowly incorporated the Weisberg Way into my life. I have been walking ever since.

In retrospect, I understand that my body never failed me but that I failed it. I ignored the obvious warning signs that had been there for a very long time. Furthermore, I neglected to do anything about it until the problem left me crippled. Once I began paying attention to the signs my body was giving me, I was able to read them and respond more appropriately. The better I served the needs of my body, the better my body served mine.

I recently had the good fortune to celebrate my 90th birthday. My family threw me an unforgettable party with wonderful company, food, and music. My greatest joy that evening was being able to *dance* with everyone there!

2: The Chair Is the Seat of All Evil

RIGHT NOW, AT THIS VERY MOMENT, you're reading this book. Perhaps it's late at night. You've just worked a long, hard day, and you're getting cozy on the couch. Or perhaps it's morning. The kids are off to school, and you've pulled up a chair at the kitchen table. Or maybe you're in your dorm, kicking back on a beanbag chair in the lounge. No matter where you are, who you are, or what time of day it is, you're probably sitting.

Sitting has become an integral part of everyday living. In all Western societies, and most Eastern ones, there are objects to sit on in virtually every room of every home. We sit in the living room, dining room, bedroom, and den. We sit at school, at work, at leisure, and sometimes even while we exercise. We sit in front of the TV, behind our desks, inside movie theaters, and outside on park benches. We sit in cars, buses, trains, planes, offices, and waiting rooms. We sit at sporting events, concerts, and parties. Life has virtually become an endless series of going from chair to chair. In fact, we perform nearly all tasks, whether for pleasure or purpose, while sitting. We are so accustomed to it that it is an act we simply take for granted. While many of us may have a vague notion that all the endless hours of sitting are somehow bad for our health, there are very few who give the physiological implications more than a moment's thought. But we can't afford to be ignorant any longer.

In the previous chapter, you learned how pervasive the problem of chronic musculoskeletal pain has become. Sadly, with each passing year, the problem gets worse. Why are there more people in pain today than ever before in history? Why is it that the number of people suffering is increasing rather than decreasing, especially when we live in an era of some of the most remarkably advanced scientific, medical, and technological achievements? Why are more and more young children hurting and alarming numbers of senior citizens nearly crippled? How is it possible that hundreds of millions of people from different countries, cultures, and classes share a common experience of chronic pain? And most perplexing of all, why are there currently whole communities whose members have almost *no* incidences of chronic pain? You might think that it would be impossible to find a single answer to all these questions, but in fact you need not look very far. You're sitting on it.

The chair is a not a new invention, but its widespread use is. While its history predates ancient Egypt, it wasn't until the mid-19th century that we became what I like to call a "sitting culture." The consequences of this drastic and sudden change in lifestyle were profound. Not only did it bring about an equally drastic change in the kind of pain from which people suffered, it also brought an equally drastic increase in the number of people who suffered. Remarkably, this correlation has been lost on a significant portion of the medical establishment. There are many in this community who contend that the modern epidemic of chronic pain is a manifestation of the human body's being inherently flawed. In their estimation, the biomechanical function and structural design of the musculoskeletal system is simply unable to withstand the effects of gravity, activity, and aging. In *The Archaeology of Disease,* a highly respected book on the subject, Keith Manchester sums up this position by stating that "one of the penalties paid by mankind for his adoption of the erect bipedal posture [walking on two feet] is his susceptibility to vertebral osteophytosis [skeletal degeneration]."[1] In other words, it is the human body that, inevitably, causes itself pain.

I wholeheartedly disagree. This "nature gone wrong" theory, as you are about to discover, ignores a whole host of evidence to the contrary. In truth, *it is not the body but rather what we do with it that causes us pain.*

Standing on Our Own Two Feet

Over the last 200 years, humanity has managed to upset what nature took millions of years of trial and error to perfect. That is because for the past two centuries most humans have participated in a daily ongoing revolution that runs counter to the evolutionary function of their bodies. Although this revolution of prolonged sitting, and the sedentary lifestyle it encourages, happens with little fanfare, it radically reduces the quality of life for hundreds of millions of people. The reason for this is simple: The biomechanical structure of the human body was not designed for chairs.

Our distant ancestors took their first upright steps nearly 4 million years ago. The theory of evolution postulates that they became bipedal as a response to external stimuli that otherwise would have threatened their survival. Walking on two feet certainly had its advantages. The early hominids were able to affect the movement of their bodies in ways that their quadrupedal ancestors could not. This flexible posture had a profound effect on this budding species. It facilitated the freedom to forage for food in unique ways, to run after prey or hide from predators more efficiently, and, eventually, with the advent of our direct ancestors, *Homo erectus,* approximately 2 million years ago, to build shelter and create tools. Walking on two feet also had a profound effect upon this species' relationship to gravity, and it was their adaptations to this that made them distinctly human.

Revolution, NOT Evolution

For them to walk on two feet and remain erect for any substantial length of time, some very important physiological adaptations had to occur. These adaptations, which eventually provided just the right amount of flexibility, stability, and vertical balance to sustain the bipedal posture, were the direct response to a shift in the center of gravity. The center of gravity, or the point at which the entirety of body weight converges (near the navel), needed to be supported appropriately so that the body could remain in equilibrium with a minimal amount of musculoskeletal effort. With the base of support or weight-bearing now falling on two extremities instead of four, evolution led to a restructuring and reorganization of the muscles and bones in the feet and ankles. It also saw a rearticulation and reangulation of the knee and hip joints and a reorientation of the pelvic tilt.

Perhaps the most important adaptation was the morphing of the spinal column from its C curvature (found in our ancestral primates and early hominids) into the unique S curvature that we have today. As bipedal posture became increasingly erect, the spinal column became increasingly straight. This is because the C curvature did not permit enough height and flexibility in stride. Furthermore, it placed the center of gravity forward so that the upper extremities needed to be used for balance and gait. But the spine did not evolve into a fixed and completely vertical structure. Rather, it developed four distinct curves to best absorb the impact of walking on two feet.

The spine is an extraordinary example of exquisite engineering design. The S curvature permits a smooth transmission of body weight directly to the legs so that the center of gravity is balanced over a vertical axis (see 2–1, page 28). It also has just the right amount of pliable bend to absorb the gravitational forces that act upon it. This means that when the curvature is maintained with optimal posture, the gravitational forces have minimal impact because they are appropriately distributed onto the structure. Furthermore, the spine, as well as the rest of the skeleton, benefits from these gravitational forces because the pulling on the bones increases their density and strength. (For more on the spine, see Chapter 3, page 64.) Although gravitational forces do compress the spine and, by extension, the protective cushions or discs that lie between the bony spinal vertebrae, it takes a long time—many hours of continuous standing—for this to occur. Remarkably, it doesn't take very long for the structural components to return to normal. All they need is a little rest.

Releasing the gravitational forces from the spine and relaxing the fatigued musculature responsible for maintaining an erect posture must happen throughout the day. When the spine is rested, it is resilient enough to absorb the impact of both walking and gravity. Without sufficient reprieves, the spinal column, in particular the lower back, will slowly but surely deteriorate. The deterioration of the spine and the deflation of the discs, in turn, reduce almost all musculoskeletal function, because the spine is the central structure around which all bodily operations revolve.

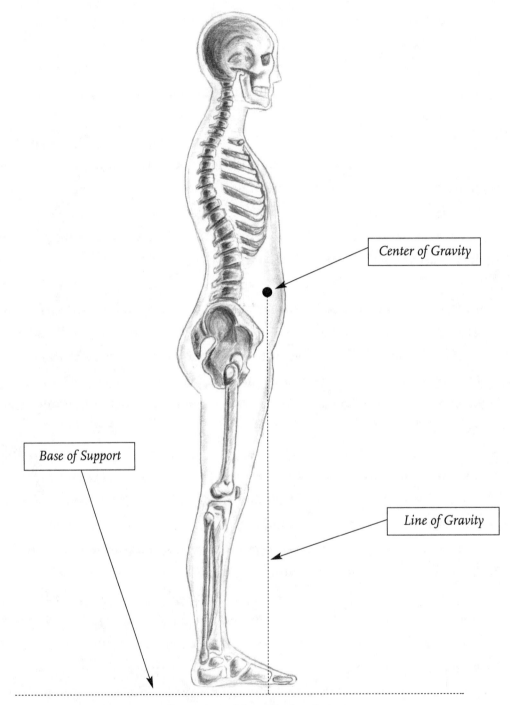

Center of Gravity

Base of Support

Line of Gravity

2–1. Illustration of the spine in relation
to the forces of gravity and the base of support

Those conditions of biomechanical dysfunction lead to a whole host of chronic pain. Fortunately, periodic respites allow the spinal column to recover from the demands of standing erect. Thus, *evolution shaped us into perfect creatures that could enjoy all of the advantages of the bipedal posture without suffering any of the disadvantages.*

But there's a catch. To counteract the potentially destructive gravitational forces, the spine must be *properly* rested. There are only two ideal ways to do this. The first is to lie down horizontally. The second method is to rest in such a way that the spine is free of downward vertical pressure while weight-bearing remains on the feet. The latter is, in a word, *squatting* (see 2–2, page 30). While the horizontal position is an effective way to let the spine rebound, it is highly impractical other than for sleep. Squatting, on the other hand, is one of the most healthy and practical ways to position the human body. This is because it completely rests the lower regions of the spine while allowing one to be alert and readily mobile at the same time. Squatting, unlike lying down, is also therapeutic, because it provides for the biological needs of additional muscle groups and joints critically affected by the maintaining of the bipedal posture. Specifically, it stretches the muscles in the back and lower extremities, thus restoring their optimal length, and takes the hips, knees, and ankles through their full range of motion, thus lubricating them with nourishing synovial fluid. Squatting, finally, is one of the most natural of bodily positions. Human toddlers squat instinctually, as do our primate cousins. And so did our ancient ancestors.

Without being aware of it, the first anatomically modern humans, the *Homo sapiens,* who appeared c. 100,000 BCE, promoted the health of their musculoskeletal systems. They were active beings who used their muscles and joints in ways that optimized their condition, such as walking to get where they were going, running to or from wild roving beasts, and climbing trees to search for food or safety. While we don't know the minute details of their everyday lives, we have a general idea of how they lived, in part from the cave paintings they left behind. These crude renderings depict the animals they hunted, the utensils they used, and the rituals and activities they participated in. Notably, these drawings from all over the world contain absolutely no images of chairs or seating objects of any kind. So what did our ancestors sit on? Nothing. They squatted. (Some ancients also sat cross-legged on

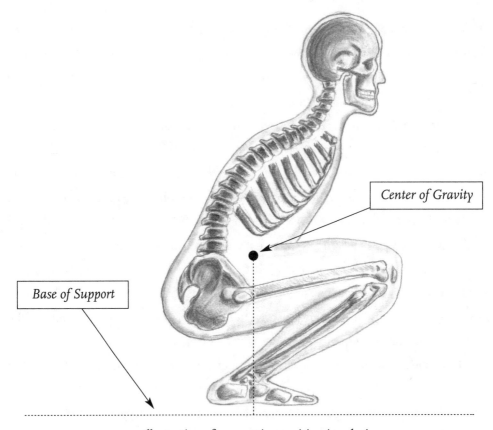

Center of Gravity

Base of Support

*2–2. Illustration of a squatting position in relation
to the forces of gravity and the base of support*

the floor. While this position has some therapeutic value in that it takes the hips and pelvis through their full range of motion and stretches some of the muscles that maintain the bipedal posture, it does not relieve the spine from the downward gravitational forces, as the structure is still vertical. However, the squatting position was also used daily: Floor-sitters had to squat at least twice a day to evacuate.) Thus these primitive prehistoric peoples engaged in a sound lifestyle that saw a balanced interplay between appropriate movement and appropriate rest.

The shift away from a rehabilitative squatting position to a debilitative sitting position parallels the shift away from hunting and gathering to agriculture. These once nomadic peoples established fixed communities with more permanent dwellings. No longer roaming from place to place, they were less mobile and more apt to accumulate belongings, most designed to accommodate a more stationary life. While there is a tendency to think that the transition from foraging to farming was a progressive and positive step in the development of civilization, it actually came at a high price.[2] With the advent of agricultural society came a sharp decline in health, including musculoskeletal health. Although the tools they created during this time (the Neolithic Era, c. 8000 to 4000 BCE) increased the efficiency of their lives in many ways, they inadvertently introduced an invention that diminished the proper use of their bodies. This invention sparked a lifestyle revolution that would both comfort and cripple much of humanity in the millennia to come.

Thrones, Moans, and Groans

Not surprisingly, the first recorded use of the chair in Egypt, c. 3100 BCE, coincides closely with the first recorded incidence of back pain in the Edwin Smith papyrus. That's because chair sitting is the most damaging, debilitating, and destructive way to position the human body. Unfortunately, it has also become the most common, but it wasn't always like this. In fact, the chair revolution started slowly.

Initially, chairs, or, more appropriately, thrones, were used almost exclusively as symbolic devices. More than providing stature, the chair highlighted particular individuals and set them apart from the group or community to which they belonged. Thus chairs were reserved for a select few to signify their position of power or religious standing. The earliest indications of the chair's special designation have been gleaned from clay figurines dating from the Neolithic period (a matrifocal era that depended upon and revered female fertility), which seem to highlight women's status by depicting them seated in chairs. Galen Cranz, in her wonderful book on the subject, appropriately titled *The Chair*, says that the early use of the chair "literally expresses high status; it separates, and elaborates the separation, providing distinction, while it legitimizes support of the occupant's whole physical and psychological being."[3]

The ushering-in of classical antiquity in Egypt saw a shift from a matrifocal to a patriarchal society, but it did little to change the symbolic use of the chair.

Here, too, chairs were used almost exclusively—as thrones—by the pharaohs and some members of the nobility. Although Egyptian craftsmen employed stools during this period and benches could be found in some dwellings, the individual chair was still the domain of a select few. While the upper echelons of society used the chair to convey a sense of status, significance, and even spirituality, it played almost no role in the daily lives of ordinary ancient men and women. Luckily for them, they continued to squat.

From the beginning, the structural design of the chair completely ignored the structural design of the human body. Symbology was favored over anatomy, and even form and function were a mere afterthought. What did the first chairs look like? Not much different from what they do today. The earliest chairs were right-angled: their flat seat pans were perpendicular to their straight backrests and parallel to the floor. While the ancient Egyptians created some variations on this design, including thrones with curved seat pans and no backrests, for the most part, the original right-angled archetype—with its upright, generally unassisted, and formal postural connotations—was preserved. But all of this changed with the birth of a new civilization.

The fifth century BCE saw a cataclysmic shift in human culture. At its epicenter in the West were the Greeks. With their insatiable appetite for learning and logic came a newfound fascination with leisure. The classical Greeks prized conversation, curiosity, and above all comfort, and these new values were reflected in the design of their chairs. Because the Greeks saw a relaxed, assisted, and informal posture as a symbol of status, they modified the Egyptian thrones by curving the backrest in a concave fashion. They also made them lighter and less bulky. Thus the creation of the Greek *clismos* marks two unique events in the history of the chair: It was the first to encourage a seated posture in the C-shaped curvature that we evolved away from, and it was the first to be domesticated.

We can thank the ancient Greeks for popularizing both slumping and chair sitting itself. Not only did they change how we sit, they also changed who did the sitting. No longer in the exclusive realm of ceremony for the rich and powerful, the *clismos* made its way into the lives of statsmen, scientists, and students alike.

The comfort and accessibility of this chair in turn affected the amount of time one spent in a seated position. While chairs were still a rare commodity by modern standards, for both the Greeks and the classical Romans who followed the era of the "sitting culture" had begun.

For the next thousand years after the fall of the Western Roman Empire in CE 476, the two types of chairs that had been fortified by the Greeks, namely, the straight backrest throne and the curved backrest *clismos,* remained virtually unchanged. As humanity slipped into the entropy of the Dark Ages, so too did the chair. The environment of political unrest, religious wars, and intellectual stagnation did little to foster the creative juices needed for innovation, especially when it came to a superfluous piece of furniture. Furthermore, the impermanent feudal home made a cumbersome and luxurious device highly expendable. Once again, the chair was reserved for a select few while the masses resumed squatting. It virtually took a backseat.

The chair began to make a comeback as humanity emerged from the Middle Ages. As peace, wealth, and enlightened ideas about the individual spread, so too did sitting in chairs. Once again, they found favor with aristocrats and courtesans, and even some important commoners were known to have more than one chair in their homes.

With trade between East and West developing, cross-cultural influences began to infiltrate chair design. Most notably, convex lumbar support created by the Chinese during the Ming Dynasty was introduced to the West. In fact, the period from the Renaissance to the mid-1800s saw the invention of all sorts of clever, task-specific, and functional chairs. Nonetheless, because they were custom- and handmade, they were expensive and scarce. It took another revolution, one that reverberated throughout the world, to accelerate the chair's widespread use.

The Industrial Revolution of the 19th century completely altered the social, political, and economic landscape. One of the most radical impacts on humanity was how swiftly it changed our relationship to the chair. For the first time in history, chairs were mass-produced, and the cost of production, both of labor and materials, was low. Their availability and affordability made chairs accessible to a whole new segment of the population: the industrial working class. As employment for this new class moved from the fields to the factories, chairs accompanied them. No longer were workers outdoors standing up; they were now indoors sitting down. With the advent of long workdays came long hours spent sitting in chairs. Once the habit of prolonged sitting was implanted in the work environment, it was only a matter of time before it made its way into the home. By the 20th century, chairs were no longer a symbol of power and prestige; they were an indispensable part of productivity and daily life. In little more than a hundred years, chairs went from being an extravagance to being a basic need.

Today, most of the global population has completely shifted from squatting to sitting in chairs. Never before in our 4-million-year history has a lifestyle transformation been incorporated into the fabric of life as abruptly. Not only did this sudden and rapid change leave our bodies absolutely no time to adapt (evolution did not have the requisite time to take the revolution into account), it also robbed us of squatting as a primary source of therapeutic rest for the musculoskeletal system. Furthermore, never before in our entire history has a human-made device as radically challenged our basic physical makeup. What is wrong with the chair's design? Why is its shape incongruous with our own? How can something so seemingly benign wreak so much havoc on the human body? The answers to these questions may shock you. Are you sitting down?

Beware the Chair

Let me start off by saying that *there are no good chairs*. There are only varying degrees of more destructive and less destructive. Ergonomic designers can tinker all they want with lumbar support, arm rests, and seat pans, but their work will be mostly in vain. No alterations can be made that will change the basic fact that right-angled chairs are bad for the body. The truth is that chairs are the single greatest and most consistent source of musculoskeletal microtraumatic injury and biomechanical dysfunction because *their* very nature goes against *ours*.

Chairs distort one of the most fundamental structures in the human body: the spine. When the unique S curvature of the spine is optimally maintained, gravitational forces are distributed appropriately onto the vertebrae. The vertebrae, in turn, appropriately compress the discs that lie between them. Thus no surface area on the structure is burdened more than any another. When the body is positioned in a right-angled chair, with the midregion of the spine flush against a backrest and the lower and upper regions bent forward, the S shape morphs into a C shape, or kyphotic curve (see 2–3, page 36). This most common sitting position is known as slumping. The loss of the S curvature, and particularly the loss of the lumbar lordosis, or lowest inward curve, causes the gravi-

Warning: Chairs are hazardous to your musculoskeletal health.

tational forces to fall more on the anterior (front) portion of the spine rather than on the posterior (back) portion. This unequal distribution overburdens both vertebrae and discs alike, because the forces fall upon areas of the structure that are not designed to withstand it. One of the most painful consequences of this is a slipped or herniated disc. Furthermore, studies have shown that it takes as few as 20 minutes for slumping to result in a loosening of the posterior spinal ligaments, which weakens the whole back.[4] With prolonged and consistent exposure to this type of postural disfigurement (which is so habitual that it infiltrates the standing posture as well), the spine begins to deteriorate and eventually erode. Even though it may take years for the damage or arthritic changes to produce symptoms, the continual microtraumatic irritation and cumulative destruction will eventually exact a price.

If you think that sitting up straight in your chair will solve the problems, think again. Whether straight or slumping, sitting in chairs puts 30 percent more pressure on the spine than standing.[5] Why does the pressure increase? Basic physics tells us that for every force there is an equal and opposite force. When you are standing, the downward gravitational forces are transmitted through the spine to the base of support at the feet while an equal and opposite force is transmitted from the feet back to the spine (see 2–1, page 28). The feet are equipped to handle this pressure (along with the entirety of body weight), but the spine is not. However, the spine is protected because the forces are diffused and absorbed as they pass through the ankles, knees, and hips on their return back. Thus the spine is subjected to only a fraction of the forces acting up on it. Chairs change the location of

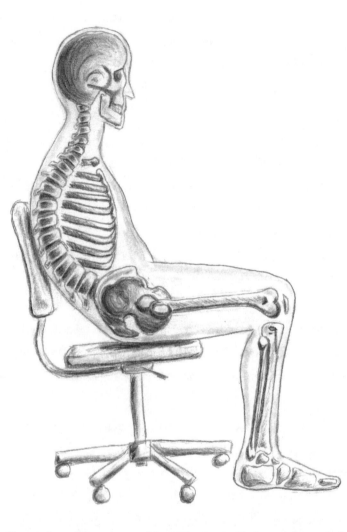

2–3. Illustration of the spine positioned kyphotically in a right-angled chair

the base of support from the feet—at the floor—to the pelvis—at the seat pan of the chair (see 2–4). The spine continues to transmit the downward gravitational forces to the base of support while you are sitting, but the pressure now falls on a base of support that is ill equipped to handle it. Likewise, the pelvis, acting in a inappropriate biomechanical and functional capacity, continues to transmit an equal and opposite force back to the spine but now without buffers to absorb it. Thus, an intense concentration of pressure coalesces in the lower back. After 45 minutes, this

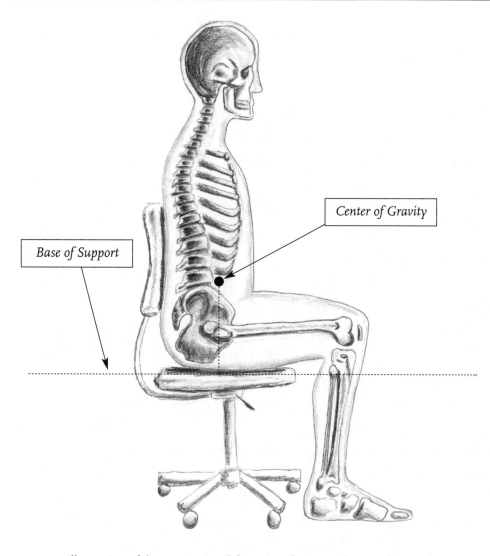

Base of Support

Center of Gravity

2–4. Illustration of the gravitational forces in relation to the seated base of support

is simply too much for an area that is already one of the most vulnerable regions in the entire body.[6] (Thus it is important to break up the duration of sitting by standing up at least once every hour.) As the lower back buckles under the incessant pressure, it causes tissue damage and pain, and prolonged consistent exposure to such microtraumatic injuries causes damage that is often permanent.

And the problems with chairs don't end there. Every time you want to sit down and take a load off, you're actually putting a load on. That's because sitting in chairs is hard work. Ironically, there is a tendency to think of sitting as a very restful position. Unfortunately, sitting rests the parts of the body that don't need much of it while working the parts that desperately do. Specifically, it disengages the lower extremities while utilizing the spine. (This is in sharp contrast to squatting, which disengages the spine while utilizing the lower extremities.) Because sitting positions the spine vertically, it provides no rest or relief from the gravitational forces that compress it. Without a periodic therapeutic reprieve through the day, the relentless load overwhelms the entire structure, joints and muscles alike. To maintain an erect seated posture, some muscle groups in the back have to continually contract. Since this requires a great deal of energy, the muscles quickly become fatigued. (That is why slumping is more comfortable: It takes less energy to maintain.) When the muscles tire, you rely on the backrest more and your muscles less. The less you rely on your muscles, the weaker and more dysfunctional they become. The weaker and more dysfunctional they become, the more you rely on the backrest. The more you rely on the backrest, the more you tend to slump. The more you slump, the more pronounced the debilitating C-shaped curvature becomes. This weakens the muscles in your back even further, which causes them to overload the joints they serve. Sitting in chairs affects even the areas seemingly at rest (particularly the hips and knees). Because sitting keeps the joints static for long periods, the muscles that serve them become fixed in a short, tight position. When at last you do get up and move, the muscles impose more stress on these joints, thereby increasing their susceptibility to wear and tear. The prolonged stasis also prevents the joints from being lubricated with nourishing synovial fluid. Once depleted, the hips and knees, like the spine, deteriorate and erode.

Is it any wonder that the areas most traumatized by sitting, namely, the lower back, hips, and knees, are also the most arthritic and disabled areas of the body in the world today? The real mystery is why so few people have made the connection between prolonged sitting and the epidemic of chronic pain. In fact, they need only look to their own bodies for an abundance of evidence.

The Chair's Legacy: Etched in Bone

All bones tell a story. They are like tablets on which the conditions of one's life are written. Their size, shape, length, strength, and density are general characteristics that reflect the environment in which one lived, the food one ate, the diseases or traumas one suffered, and the physical activities that filled one's days. Structural abnormalities or arthritic changes are particularly revealing because the deviations reflect unique events that happened to an individual. Specifically, these modifications indicate unusual stress or irritation that were severe or frequent enough to cause the bone to change. The comparative study of skeletons from primitive cultures, both ancient and modern, with those from contemporary cultures, including the present day, provides tangible pieces of additional proof that evolution went right and our lifestyle revolution went terribly wrong.

For close to 2 million years, all human beings have shared the same basic anatomy. If we are to believe those who say that walking on two feet is an engineering disaster that is responsible for the epidemic of chronic pain, we would expect to find a uniform and similar pattern of arthritis in all peoples throughout history. We would expect gender, age, and cultural norms and habits to play but a small role, with the human condition itself playing the largest role in bringing about arthritic changes.

In fact, we have found that the opposite is true. According to the bioarcheologist Clark Spenser Larsen, "Osteoarthritis is highly revealing about lifestyle and workload. Although the disorder is somewhat influenced by climate, genetics, and other factors, it is workload and physical activity—what bioarcheologists call the mechanical environment—that best explains the presence of OA."[7] For instance, ancient male bones from the Great Basin area in North America show a high degree of severe arthritis in the feet and ankles. This was not from flawed anatomy but because they were hunters who had to travel over demanding terrain for long distances to find suitable sources of prey. Ancient female bones from Patuxent Point in Europe show severe arthritis in the elbows and hands because of gender-specific work-related tasks particular to their society.[8] In areas where spear hunting was prevalent, we see more arthritis in the shoulders. In cultures where fishing was common, we see more arthritis in the shoulders, elbows, and hands.[9] In other words, it was extreme conditions and functional abuse—not ordinary and general use—that caused these pathologies. The presence of rampant arthritis in specific areas of ancient skeletons and the absence of any degree of uniformity between cultures tells us that the degeneration was a result of individual sociology, *not* universal biology.

Because specific lifestyle choices determine the type, locale, and severity of arthritic changes and pain one suffers from, we should see arthritis express itself differently in bones sampled from primitive cultures and from modern ones. Guess what? We do. Skeletal remains from the Paleolithic era (200,000 to 10,000 BCE) are riddled with arthritis, yet the locations of abnormalities are as varied as the specimens examined. In fact, the skeletons are able to assist in painting a clear picture of ancient daily life because the arthritic degeneration is so individualized.

This is in sharp contrast to modern bone specimens, which, in spite of being taken from all over the world, show a uniformity of arthritis for the first time in history. For example, the World Health Organization (WHO) reports that the joints most frequently affected by osteoarthritis today are the knees, hips, and spine. In the United States alone, knee and hip OA together account for more lower-extremity disability than any other disease.[10] The WHO also reports that 75 percent to 85 percent of the total global population will experience arthritis-related back pain at some time in their lives. Although the prevalence of culturally specific arthritis in other anatomical areas still exists, the uncanny similarity in arthritic patterns in almost all peoples happened only within the past 150 years. According to Edward Shorter of the faculty of medicine of the University of Toronto, "Patients presenting with chronic lower-back pain are historically new patients, in the sense that they did not exist in distant times."[11] While lower-back pain isn't a recent condition—for instance, the ancient Hippocratic writings of the classical Greeks contain treatments for lower-back pain as a result of kyphosis[12]—the epidemic proportions of the outbreak and the uniformity of chronic pain is a uniquely modern phenomenon. Because this phenomenon is common to the diverse and exceedingly large worldwide population, it must have a common cause.

Since arthritic patterns have eliminated evolutionary flaws as the culprit and implicated lifestyle instead, what is the collective thread that causes this uniformity of chronic pain to occur? What affects the knees, hips, and spine to such a degree that it leads to the frequency of arthritis we see today, especially when these pathologies were rarities in our ancestors? What do we have that they didn't? The answer to all of these questions is, of course, the chair.

Some of the most illuminating evidence demonstrating the link between the chair and chronic pain comes not from people who have arthritis but from those who don't. In a landmark study of Indian jungle dwellers, the noted orthopedic researcher W. Harry Fahrni found this population to have only a 9 percent incidence of lumbar disc degeneration, as opposed to 35 percent found in a comparative study of European office personnel. He also found that the Indians had "an almost zero incidence of back pain."[13] Ongoing orthopedic studies of the geographic and ethnic differences in the prevalence of global arthritis found that "OA of the hip is least common in Japanese, Saudi Arabian, Chinese, and African populations."[14] What explains these findings? What do such diversified peoples have in common that excludes them from exhibiting the uniformity of arthritis that their contemporary peers display? Or, more accurately, what don't they have that others do? Once again, the answer is the chair.

Specifically, our contemporaries who do not exhibit a uniformity of arthritis come from squatting, not chair sitting, cultures. According to Fahrni and Gordon Trueman, "On the basis of radiographic studies [X-rays], the incidence of degenerative change in the intervertebral discs in squatting populations is considerably less than that found in [other] peoples."[15] The German researcher T. Hettinger supports this conclusion in that "two populations of Africans and Asians who squat rather than sit on chairs report far less compression of the spine than do Europeans doing either light *or* heavy work."[16] (Emphasis added.) And Donald Gunn, a distinguished orthopedic surgeon and lecturer at Tan Tock Seng Hospital in Singapore, attributes the rarity of primary OA in the hips of Asians to their habit of squatting and sitting cross-legged on the floor.[17] Thus the elimination of the abnormal forces that the chair imposes on the body coupled with the inclusion of therapeutic movement (squatting) directly influences the ability to maintain optimal musculoskeletal health.

Chairs Are Here to Stay

We can no more function without chairs than we can without cars and telephones. Does this mean that we are doomed to live with crippling arthritis and chronic pain? Absolutely not. I am not suggesting that we get rid of chairs or even that we need to so that we can live a pain-free life. The important lesson to learn from the damaging skeletal evidence indicting chairs is that bodily preservation must be based on complementing our evolutionary biomechanical design while minimizing the consequences of our revolutionary lifestyle. In other words, painful conditions are not the result of things outside of our control, such as our physiological makeup, but rather are caused by things within our sphere of control, such as our habits. Therefore, *it's time to stop blaming our bodies. Instead, it's time to start taking care of them.*

How do we take care of our bodies? Ancient bones indicate that musculoskeletal pain used to be almost entirely a result of disease, diet (specifically, from the lack of calcium), or macrotraumas (including injuries from overuse). Our modern technology and science have all but eliminated these factors as the primary sources of musculoskeletal pain: Many bone diseases are preventable or treatable, diet has been vastly improved, and macrotraumatic injuries can be properly healed. The final frontier then is to counteract the microtraumatic damage caused by sitting in chairs. And that's exactly what the Weisberg Way is designed to do. The 3-Minute Maintenance Method uses six specially designed therapeutic movements, including the Natural Squat, to protect the muscles and joints that are most at risk from prolonged sitting. Specifically, it heals microtraumas, restores biomechanical function, and makes the musculoskeletal system more resistant to wear and tear by providing for its biological needs on a daily basis. My program also counteracts the other big problem that prolonged chair sitting causes: the deficiency of movement.

We are all guilty of being couch potatoes to some extent. Whether watching movies or staring at computer screens, we spend most of our time sitting. This means that we don't spend a lot of time moving. It is important to understand that chairs are only one piece of the chronic-pain puzzle. Another giant piece is the sedentary lifestyle they encourage. In the final analysis, the chair's most dangerous legacy may be the deficiency of movement, because it is responsible for staggering amounts of arthritis and chronic pain. If you want to know why this deficiency is so bad and how my program is able to make it better, pull up a chair (if you dare!) and read on.

Happy Endings: Mike's Story

Mike A., age 38, is a film director, screenwriter, and four-time Jeopardy! *champion. He is also an expert theatrical swordsman who injured his L$_3$ vertebra in his back while performing a fight in a stunt show more than 15 years ago.*

My name is Mike, and I am a recovering ergonomics chair junky. I developed an addiction to these contraptions approximately five years after I injured my back. Although it only took a few months for the initial injury to heal, within a few years, back pain had become a constant in my life. Until then, I never realized how much time I spent sitting. Because I was unable to sit without it hurting, I went searching for the perfect chair. Sparing no expense, I purchased every conceivable ergonomic chair on the market. I bought one for every room of my apartment and one for my office. Some had stationary lumbar rolls; others had movable lumbar rolls. Some had high back support; others had no back support at all. Remember kneeling chairs? I had one of those too. Eventually I added adjustable armrests, then adjustable neck rests, and finally adjustable foot rests. I even bought weird-looking inflatable portable devices that would make any chair ergonomically correct. I knew I had hit bottom when some, such as stools, perches, and zero-gravity seats, didn't resemble chairs at all. Did any of them fix my problem? No. In fact, to my shock and dismay, my pain only got worse.

I learned from Dr. Weisberg that my desperate search for the perfect chair was futile. There are no perfect chairs. It doesn't matter how many lumps, bumps, and extraneous gadgets the chair has, nor does it matter how much it costs. Prolonged sitting—not the type of chair you sit in—is harmful to the body, whether, like me, you've had an injury or not. Indeed, I have come to understand that habitual sitting played a major role in causing my pain relapses. Once I knew that the chair was a big part of my problem, I stopped looking for one to provide a solution.

While I do sometimes sit in an ergonomic chair, I buy only regular chairs now. If I feel that I'm missing extra support, Dr. Weisberg showed me how to use cheap household items in place of expensive ergonomic add-on (see page 193). He also told me that I should never sit for more than 45 minutes at a time without getting up, moving around, and stretching. That one piece of advice, coupled with the Weisberg Way, has cured my chair addiction and turned my painful life into a pain-free one.

3: If It's Physical, It's Therapy

IF YOU LOOK AT THE WORLD, you will see that every living thing is in motion, whether on land, in the air, or in water. Fish swim, jellyfish bob, birds fly, cats scamper, dogs jump, spiders spin their webs, and bees make honey, all in the never-ending dance of life. Every organism is designed to move in a specific way, and every organism needs movement to sustain itself. Human beings are no different. What distinguishes us from every other creature is analytic choice. Whereas the majority of organisms on earth move in response to external environmental factors, such as the wind or water currents, or internal factors, such as instinct, we are able to choose when, how, and even if we move. Unfortunately, we often choose our movements poorly without knowing why. But it wasn't always this way. We were once a species whose very survival depended on the extent to which we were able to move. While modern inventions have rendered that dependency all but obsolete, our primordial need to move remains. Our physical makeup, virtually unchanged in 10,000 years, simply has not caught up with the recent and radical shift in our lifestyle. We are in essence cavemen cloaked in modernity. As you are about to see, this incongruity is what causes the vast majority of the aches and pain from which we suffer.

We were created to move. If the great philosopher Descartes had said, "I move, therefore I am," he couldn't have been more correct, at least from a physiological standpoint. Our anatomy is specifically designed to permit and facilitate movement, and it, in turn, *requires and depends upon movement for its own preservation*. Why is this so? One of the core principles of biology is that the body will accommodate itself to the demands placed upon it. The greater the demand, the greater the body's responsiveness to meet that demand.

Movement individually stimulates all the disparate biological systems, triggering a chain of events whereby they work together to sustain life. For instance, the cardiovascular system responds to movement by stimulating the heart to beat faster, thus accelerating the rate at which blood is pumped into circulation. The circulatory system responds with an increased interaction between blood and the tissues it feeds. Thus more oxygen is brought to the organs, increasing their energy, vitality, and general life force. The digestive system responds by permitting a quicker nutritional absorption rate and a higher degree of disposal (rather than storage) of fats. The neurological system responds with enhanced alertness. The musculoskeletal system responds to movement by creating stronger, more durable, and more flexible biomechanical parts.

Since most of us lead sedentary lives, I wish I could tell you that a deficiency of movement has little effect on the body. Unfortunately, I cannot. In June 2002, the United States government released a report that attributes 300,000 deaths a year to a sedentary lifestyle.[1] Immobility causes the aforementioned processes to slow down and eventually to shut down altogether. Every system in the human body is adversely affected by lack of movement. The absence of demand causes the heart to weaken and beat less efficiently. Thus it needs to work harder to accomplish the same tasks and eventually permanently breaks down. Less blood is circulated. When oxygen distribution is reduced, the tissues of the body atrophy. Proper diges-

Lack of Movement = The 4 Ds:

Dysfunction, Decay, Disease, Death

tion is impaired, and deposits of fat form. Weight gain and obesity occur, which inhibit mobility even further. Muscles become weak, and joints become stiff, arthritic, and painful. The only way to avoid this is to move. But there's a catch. If simply getting up and moving (which is inevitable at some point) or even exercising were enough to sufficiently facilitate health, everyone would be healthy. This is obviously not the case. In fact, moving under less than optimal conditions can actually cause problems rather than solve them. This is where my program comes in. The Weisberg Way is designed to bridge the gap between our lifestyle and our biological needs. It uses the curative value of movement to supplement the discrepancy between what we demand *of* our bodies and what our bodies demand *from* us in return. To understand how my program works, you first need to get reacquainted with something very near and dear to you: your own anatomy.

The human body is an extraordinary living machine. The more I learn about it (and I still learn something new and fascinating almost every day), the more I am humbled by its infinite wonders. It can literally take volumes to explain the subtle complexities of the human body. That is not my purpose here. What I will focus on are the aspects of anatomy that relate directly to movement, that is, the components of the musculoskeletal system. Why? Because the body as a whole can benefit only when the individual elements that enable movement are sustained in optimal health; to keep these elements healthy one must become acquainted with the mechanics of how they work. Toward that end I will introduce you to the mechanics of your skeletal system, including your bones, joints, joint capsules, cartilage, and ligaments; your muscular system, including your muscles and tendons; and your spinal column.

The Skeletal System

What kind of creature would you be without your skeleton? Nothing more than a formless heap of tissues and organs. The *skeletal system* provides the foundation on which the human body is built. It is the living, dynamic framework that functions, much like a clothes hanger, to shape and support your entire structure. It also protects vital organs and acts as an anchor for the muscles that move it. The skeleton is made up of more than 200 *bones*, which are linked together at over 100 movable *joints*. Other components of the skeletal system include *cartilage* and *ligaments*.

Bones

ANATOMICAL DESCRIPTION Bones are active, springy, and resilient organs that are in a constant state of growth, remodeling, and repair. They are a storehouse for calcium and other minerals and are dynamically involved in their transfer to and supply of the rest of the body. Some bones participate in the building of the immune system by producing (in the bone marrow) red and white blood cells. Most important for our purposes, bones are very strong and are tough enough to withstand the constant stress and load that bears down on them yet sufficiently light enough to easily enable movement.

In an adult human there are typically 206 bones that come in a remarkable variety of shapes and sizes. The unique dimension and constitution of each bone perfectly matches its function. For instance, the long bones of the arms and legs function to withstand both the vertical and horizontal forces of compression that constantly work on them. The flat bones of the shoulders and hips function to provide a sizable surface area for the muscles of comparable size that anchor or attach to them. And the rounded nature of the pelvis and rib cage function to protect the fragile occupants (intestines and heart, among them) that lie within. Some bones are movable, such as those found in the hands and feet, and some are immobile, such as those found in the skull. All bones have a dense outer layer, which accounts for their strength, and a spongelike inner layer, which accounts for their reduced weight. If not for this paradoxical microstructure, bones would restrict rather than permit movement.

Bone is a type of connective tissue, or bundle of specialized cells, that is surrounded by a substance called a matrix. The matrix is composed chiefly of two elements that work in complementary ways: protein, which makes bone supple, and calcium, which makes it immalleable. The architecture of bone is not completely fixed; it is rather in a continuous flux of breaking down and rebuilding. How is this possible? Inside the matrix live two types of cells: osteoblasts and osteoclasts. Osteoblasts build bone by producing new cells and depositing protein and calcium on its surface. At the same time, osteoclasts erode bone by breaking down old cells and diverting protein and calcium to other parts of the body. These two oppositional yet balancing processes adjust according to the needs and demands placed on the body.

BIOLOGICAL NEEDS Healthy bones can last for more than 120 years! They achieve their long-lasting durability through movement. Movement is essential for their optimal upkeep for two very important reasons: It increases calcium depository and it stimulates new bone production. Let's look at each of these vital processes individually.

Bone is made up primarily of calcium and therefore depends upon calcium for its health. Calcium enters the bloodstream through diet and serves multiple metabolic functions, not the least of which is the maintenance of bone tissue. Once calcium enters the body, bone will absorb as much of it as it perceives it needs. This perception accurately reflects the demands placed upon it. When you move, stress is applied to bones both externally, by gravity, and internally, by the force of muscle activity. Bones respond to this stress with an increased need for calcium. To accommodate itself to the intensified need, the body diverts more calcium to the bones that are under stress. The greater the demand, the more calcium will be diverted to them. The more calcium deposited, the stronger and more vital the bones.

Movement also increases new bone production. Under the stress of movement, bones respond by sending a signal to the osteoblasts that live on their inner and outer surfaces to build more bone. At the same time, they send a signal to shut down the function of the osteoclasts to erode bone. Thus bone mass increases at the site under stress, and the local area becomes thicker and stronger. To benefit optimally, bones need to be stressed in the most rehabilitative and advantageous way possible. There is a delicate balance that must be struck between applying enough force to stimulate change and applying too much, which can cause injury. The rate at which bone production increases is dependent on finding just the right combination between too little and too much force, which is exactly what my therapeutic movements are designed to do. In addition, movement also ensures that the bones that incur the most daily wear and tear are in a constant state of renewal and rebuilding.

As important as it is to understand how meeting the biological needs of your bones facilitates their health, it is equally important to understand how *not* meeting those needs causes bone degeneration. In bone production, lack of movement sets in motion the opposite processes from the ones mentioned above. Bone production by the osteoblasts is shut down, and bone erosion by the osteoclasts is sped up. Things go from bad to worse when it comes to calcium. Immobility creates a reduced need for calcium in the bones. Instead of the calcium's being diverted to the bones, the body excretes it as waste. What's more, the calcium stored in the bone itself is perceived as excess. Instead of holding on to their storehouse of calcium, bones release it into the bloodstream, where it too is excreted as waste. As the surplus becomes a deficit, bones grow thin and degrade. A whole host of dysfunction and disease ensues, one of them the crippling effects of osteoporosis. Now, isn't it easy to see why movement is not just important but absolutely imperative to the health of your bones?

Joints

ANATOMICAL DESCRIPTION Joints are an absolute marvel of engineering design. They are also some of the most useful components of our physiological makeup, for they are the well from which all movement springs. If the various bones of the skeleton were fused together to form one long continuous structure, it would be utterly impossible to move. To enable flexible yet stabile motion, the ends of bones do not touch; rather, they meet up at a junction, or joint. A joint is not a singular piece of anatomy. The word refers to the site where bones connect to the many anatomical elements that participate in movement (see 3–1). These elements work together synergistically to form the structural cooperative we call a joint.

Joints function in two divergent yet complementary ways. While they permit the mobility of the skeletal structure, they also restrict its movement to a prescribed range and direction. The freedom they facilitate allows for us to move in

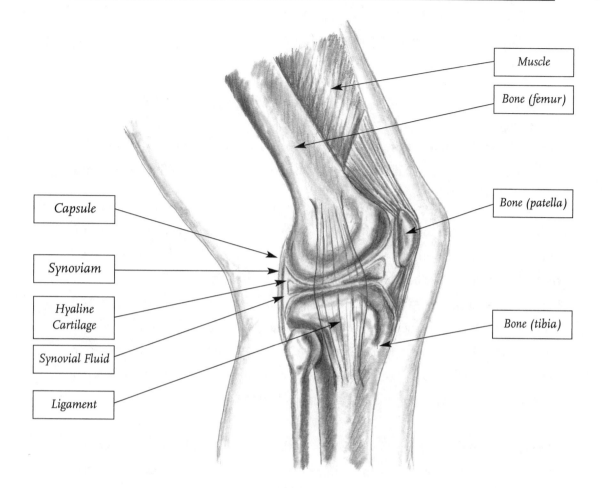

Muscle

Bone (femur)

Bone (patella)

Capsule

Synoviam

Hyaline
Cartilage

Synovial Fluid

Ligament

Bone (tibia)

3–1. Illustration of a synovial joint

an infinite variety of ways, while the limitation they impose prevents us from being nothing more than floppy rag dolls. The constant interplay between mobility and stability is determined by the unique nature of individual joints. There are more than 400 separate joints in the human body. All fall into one of three categories, and their structure determines their function: fixed joints, slightly movable joints, and synovial or movable joints.

Fixed joints are the rarest of the three. They are connected by interlocking fibrous tissue and permit only the slightest (almost imperceptible) movement. Mostly found in the skull, they secure the region by forming sutures that practically fuse the adjoining bones together. The inflexibility of these joints functions to give the skull its great strength.

Slightly movable joints make up about a third of the body's joints. Allowing more movement than fixed joints, they also limit and restrict it. For instance, some of the joints of the spine are only slightly movable, as are some of the joints found in the lower regions of the leg. The relative flexibility of these joints functions to provide the body with controlled agility.

Synovial or movable joints are the most common and most relevant for our purposes because they enable the widest range of movement. In fact, every time I mention joints in this book I am referring to synovial joints.

Synovial or movable joints are highly mechanical in nature and act as hinges and shock absorbers for the bones they adjoin. The endless variety of tasks we are able to accomplish, from the delicate and intricate movements required by the hands of a surgeon to the bold gymnastic movements required by the legs of a ballet dancer, are all made possible by synovial joints.

Joints are like pieces of a jigsaw puzzle, with the two ends of adjoining bones being the interlocking pieces. The manner in which the bones fit together determines the kind of joint they create and the freedom of movement they allow. There are six main types of synovial joints, each of which permits a specific type of motion. *Pivot joints* occur where one bone has a protrusion that fits into a pocket of another. These joints allow for a limited pivot or rotating motion, such as turning your head. *Ellipsoidal joints* are formed when an oval dome from one bone fits into the recess of another. This allows for up, down, and side-to-side motion, such as that at the base of your fingers. *Ball-and-socket joints* contain a bone with a ball-like head that fits into a compatible socket. These joints facilitate a broader range of motion than any other in the body and are found in the hip and shoulder. *Saddle joints* have bones that fit together like a pair of curved saddles. They allow for wide rotation and are found in only one place: where the thumb adjoins the hand. *Hinge joints* have one bone that rotates within a cylindrical recess. These allow for simple motion, such as bending down or straightening up, and are found in the knees and elbows. *Plane joints* contain bones with flat surfaces. These joints have extremely limited motion and are located in the foot and collarbone. Yet no matter how different the various synovial joints are from one another, their purpose is the same: to hold bones close together while permitting smooth, coordinated movement.

BIOLOGICAL NEEDS Joints are highly resilient yet incur a remarkable amount of daily wear and tear. Because they are the fundamental component in the biomechanics of movement, preserving their functionality is of utmost importance. Without proper care, they are extremely vulnerable to microtraumatic, or imperceptibly small, injuries. As I've said, the accumulation of these microscopic injuries can lead to the most catastrophic, crippling, and chronically disabling ailments. If the biomechanical condition of the joint remains poor, microtraumas will continue to wreak their havoc upon the structure. If the biomechanical condition is well maintained, microtraumas will heal and the joint's health will be sustained for a lifetime.

To prepare joints for the unique movement they permit, they need to be moved through one extreme end of their range of motion to the other daily. Because joints are an amalgam of different anatomical elements, when we talk about their needs, we are really talking about the needs of those individual components. In addition to the anatomy of the skeletal system, synovial joints also depend on elements of the *muscular system* for their health. To fully understand how to keep synovial joints in optimal condition, we will now look at each of these elements in depth.

Joint Capsule

ANATOMICAL DESCRIPTION All of the various anatomical elements that make up a synovial joint are held firmly in place by connective tissue called a joint capsule. These very strong fibers attach to the ends of the bones that meet up within the joint. The capsule encloses the entirety of the joint and connects one bone to another. Thus it gives the joint its stability, preventing any deviation from its normal range of motion while still permitting flexible movement.

The interior of the joint capsule is lined with a membrane called the *synovium*. The synovium secretes *synovial fluid*, which functions in two fundamentally important ways: It lubricates the joint for the purpose of diminishing friction, and it nourishes the surface cells of *cartilage*. The joint capsule gains additional support from *ligaments*, which connect bones, and *tendons*, which affix muscles to bones.

BIOLOGICAL NEEDS Every joint is held together by a joint capsule, and every joint capsule has a unique shape and size that is perfectly tailored for the joint it serves. To maintain its appropriate dimension, it needs to be moved through its full range of motion daily. Here's why:

The joint capsule is made up of woven connective tissue. This tissue is responsive to the demands placed upon it and will rearrange itself according to those demands. If it is not challenged or moved to its extreme range, it will tighten up and retract. This restricts the normal movement of the joint, which sets in motion a destructive chain of events, such as arthritis, that can lead to severe pain and dysfunction. Likewise, if the joint capsule is overchallenged, it loosens and elongates. This promotes instability in the joint by allowing movement beyond the scope of its normal range. This can also lead to severe dysfunction. By regularly taking the joint to both ends of its extreme range, the capsule weave retains its proper proportions. Maintaining the normal dimensions of the joint capsule facilitates its complementary service to the joint. In addition, by moving the joint through its entire range of motion, you stimulate the synovium to produce synovial fluid and ensure its equal distribution over the entire surface area of the joint's cartilage.

Cartilage

ANATOMICAL DESCRIPTION Cartilage is a resilient, spongy type of connective tissue. While its makeup, which is chiefly protein, is similar to that of bones, it is softer and more flexible. Found all over the body, cartilage comes in three main types: *elastic cartilage*, which is located in the nose and ears; *fibrocartilage*, which is located in the discs between the vertebrae in the spinal cord; and *hyaline cartilage*, which covers the ends of bones in the synovial joints. Because hyaline cartilage is one of the most significant determinant factors in the health of your joints, it demands a closer look.

When two or more movable bones come together in a joint, they easily glide across each other during movement. Hyaline cartilage makes this possible by wrapping around or capping the ends of bones, thus providing them with a smooth, slick covering. It creates an almost frictionless environment in which the bones can pivot or rotate with a minimal amount of wear and tear. Without hyaline cartilage, the ends of bones would grind against each other and erode.

Hyaline cartilage also acts as a shock absorber and cushions the bone from sudden stress and impact. In essence, it works like a sponge. Every time you move, pressure is applied to the joints that are in motion. Walking, for instance, places a force equal to three times your body weight on the involved joints. Under this force, tissue fluid, comprised of mostly water and proteins, is squeezed out of the cartilage and into the cavity between the neighboring bones. The fluid from the tissue absorbs the brunt of the impact and disperses the remainder onto the bone in an equalized fashion. When the force is released, the cartilage reabsorbs the fluid, storing it until it is needed. This process is performed an infinite number of times on any given day.

BIOLOGICAL NEEDS You begin to get a really good sense of the synergy at work among the different elements of a joint when you look at maintaining the health of cartilage. Because hyaline cartilage is under constant compression, the circulatory system does not extend to the cells of its top layer. Blood vessels are simply too delicate to withstand the forces at work here. So how does hyaline cartilage receive its nourishment? Nature, in its infinite wisdom, has taken care of this problem. The cartilage receives its nourishment from the synovial fluid produced by the joint capsule. Movement stimulates the secretion of synovial fluid in the joint capsule and also acts as its vehicle of dispersment to the hyaline cartilage. In order for cartilage to remain vital and robust, its entire surface must be exposed to synovial fluid. To ensure full exposure, the joint must be moved from one extreme end of its range of motion to the other daily.

Any portion of hyaline cartilage not in contact with synovial fluid is highly susceptible to microtraumatic injury. If the cells are deprived of nourishment, they will deteriorate and eventually die. When this happens, cartilage loses its ability to cushion bones from the stress associated with daily wear and tear. Under these conditions, bones grate against each other and the impact of movement is felt. Joints become stiff and inflamed. Bones respond by developing disfiguring protrusions. All the while, pain ensues. Pain compounds the problem because when you feel it, you move less. The less you move, the less synovial fluid reaches the cartilage. The less fluid reaches the cartilage, the more degeneration of cartilage incurs. The more degeneration, the more pain. This vicious cycle is more commonly known as arthritis.

Arthritis (not caused by disease) is a preventable condition. I'm sure that this is good news to the hundreds of millions of sufferers around the world. I will address this condition in greater detail in Chapter 7. For now it is important to understand that arthritis is a manifestation of the underlying lack of maintenance and upkeep of the hyaline cartilage. That's the problem. The solution is to maintain the health of your cartilage by taking your joints through a series of specially designed therapeutic movements once a day. This ensures that the entire cartilage surface area is bathed in healing and nutritious synovial fluid.

Ligaments

ANATOMICAL DESCRIPTION Ligaments are tough connective tissue that bind together two adjoining bones in a joint. They are made of densely packed fibers that are woven in such a way as to permit the joint to move freely. Their main function is to impose limitations on the joint by restricting its movement to the degree for which it was designed.

Ligaments are found both inside and outside the joint capsule. Their consistency and flexibility varies; some are elastic; others are quite rigid. Irrespective of location or makeup, they provide additional reinforcement and stability to the entire joint structure. Ligaments are very strong; in fact, their strength is greater than that of steel. And ligaments are extremely hard to stretch. In fact, it requires a great deal of stress to elongate them to the point of injury, what is known as a sprain. Because of their great capacity to withstand a variety of impacts and burdens, they not only hold bones together but also keep them from being dislocated or pulled apart.

BIOLOGICAL NEEDS Ligaments are similar in both structure and function to joint capsules. Thicker, more ropelike, and without synovium, they nevertheless have almost identical biological needs. Every joint has an accompanying set of ligaments, and every set of ligaments, just like joint capsules, has unique dimensions that are perfectly tailored to the joint it serves. Also like joint capsules, the woven tissues of ligaments rearrange themselves according to the demands placed on them. Too little demand causes a restriction of movement at the joint; too much demand causes instability within it. For a ligament to maintain its integrity and normal function, the tissues must remain in their prescribed shape and size. Once again, this is accomplished by moving the joint through its full range of motion daily.

The Muscular System

The skeletal system provides the flexible framework that facilitates movement; the *muscular system* provides the power. *Muscles* are vigorous, potent organs that generate enormous amounts of energy. In total they account for more than half the body's weight and are responsible for producing all movement. There are three main types of muscle tissue: *cardiac* and *smooth muscles,* found in the heart and internal organs, respectively, are involuntary and automatic; *skeletal muscles,* located throughout the body, are voluntary and respond directly to our will. Skeletal muscles taper at the ends into *tendons,* which anchor them firmly to bones.

Muscles

ANATOMICAL DESCRIPTION Muscles are the stuff of life. They protect your vital organs, keep your heart pumping, and provide the basis of interaction with the elements that make it possible for you to survive and thrive. If you were to strip away your body's surface layers of skin and fat, you would find mostly muscle. Indeed, there are more than 650 skeletal muscles alone, which range in size from tiny, such as the ones found in your ears, to massive, such as the ones found in your shoulders. No matter their size, their purpose is the same: Skeletal muscles are responsible for producing movement. And they move you by doing one thing: pulling.

Although skeletal muscles are highly complex in nature, the way they facilitate movement is actually quite simple. Skeletal muscles are attached to bones by their tough, fibrous ends, or tendons, that link two bones together across a movable joint. Because they are voluntary, they respond to electrical impulses sent from the brain. The structure of skeletal muscles is such that this neurological stimulation induces a contraction. When muscles contract, they shorten. The net effect of this change in muscular length is a pulling on the bones in the same direction as the contraction. Thus movement occurs.

Sound simple? Well, it is and it isn't. Skeletal muscles are well-adapted, highly organized, and complicated organs. They are made up of densely packed cylindrical groups of long cells known as muscle *fibers* (see Figure 3–2). Each fiber is filled with smaller fibers called *myofibrils,* and each myofibril is made up of hundreds of even smaller fibers called *myofilaments.* Myofilaments are both thick and thin and are where muscle contraction takes place. When a muscle is in a relaxed position, the thick and thin myofilaments overlap slightly. When an electrical impulse sent from the brain down through the spinal column and into the nerves dispersed within the muscle fibers arrives, the thick filaments slide between the thin filaments. (If you slide the fingers from one hand in between the fingers of the other, you will have a pretty good idea of how this system works.) As the filaments draw closer and interlace, the entire muscle fiber shortens. The more shortened the muscle fiber becomes, the greater the contraction or pulling and thus the greater the movement. When the electrical stimulation subsides, the myofilaments release the contraction, and the muscle assumes a relaxed position. The muscle will remain like this until it is again called upon to perform its function.

Skeletal muscles give new meaning to the word teamwork, because for

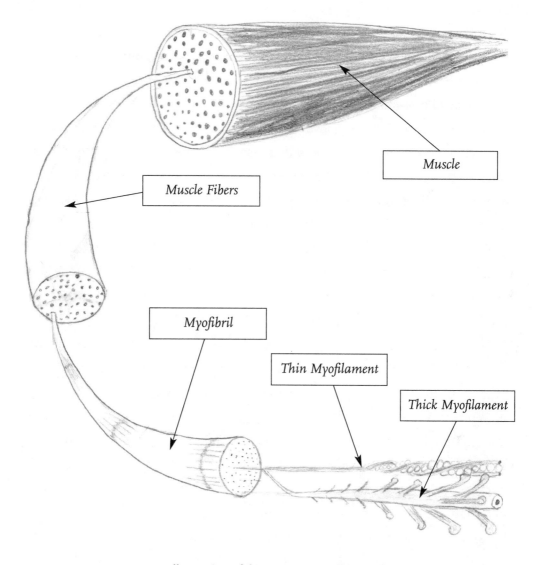

Muscle

Muscle Fibers

Myofibril

Thin Myofilament

Thick Myofilament

3–2. Illustration of the cross section of a muscle

every movement you make, two or more must work together to make it happen. As muscles have the ability to pull only the bones they adjoin, to enable a variety of movements they are arranged into oppositional, complementary pairs. As one muscle contracts and pulls on the bone, the other relaxes and ceases to pull on it. For example, when your hand brings an object close to your body, your biceps contracts and your triceps relaxes. When you push an object away from your body, you actually cause the triceps to contract and the biceps to relax. Whatever the motion, one antagonistic muscle contracts and exerts its pulling force onto the bone while its opposite relaxes and lets go of the bone. There is thus a perfect symmetry and balance to all movement.

The entire business of moving is a very costly one. Every contraction requires the production of tremendous amounts of energy. Where does the fuel come from? Muscle fibers have the unique ability to convert nutrients loaded with chemical energy into kinetic, or movement, energy. This remarkable transformation takes place during respiration when glucose is delivered to the muscles through the numerous capillaries that reside in their fibers. Glucose is then broken down by oxygen, which releases enough energy to make adenosine triphosphate (ATP). ATP is the substance that carries this newly created energy to the places where it is most needed, providing the muscles with the power they require to move.

Muscles are gas-guzzlers, yet the human body is an energy conservationist at heart. To resolve this paradox, skeletal muscles are hot-wired to use the fuel they produce in the most efficient way possible. How? There are no neutral muscle movements. Every conceivable one requires a contraction to occur, and every contraction needs a constant flow of energy to sustain it. To conserve energy, muscles automatically build physiological *bridges* across the myofilaments during a contraction. These bridges act much like glue in that they temporarily fix the muscles into contracted or shortened positions. By locking the myofilaments in place, the bridges eliminate the need to continuously refuel the contraction. Thus the consumption of energy is effectively shut down. When held in one place for a prolonged time, muscles become biochemically and electrically silent and the bridges become more permanently affixed. This shortened version is released when the position of the muscles is changed. Under optimal health conditions, the old bridges detach and new ones reattach to sustain the new position.

With the multiple operations involved in making a single movement, you might think that even the simplest motion would take an incredibly long time. Of course, this is not true. All of these processes happen in a fraction of a second. In a sense, human beings move on autopilot. The repeated exposure to everyday activities, such as walking, is infused into the deep recesses of memory. The brain auto-matically controls the muscles required for these movements, so that by the time you are conscious of wanting to move, you're already in motion. In fact, muscles themselves have a sort of memory that works much like a reflex. This is how, for in-stance, your arm instinctively goes up without a moment's thought to protect your face from an object thrown at it. It is only in trying to learn a new skill, such as play-ing the guitar, that you become fully aware of the elaborate coordination involved in muscle movement.

BIOLOGICAL NEEDS Skeletal muscles cater to your every whim. They are rugged, resilient, and highly reparative organs that are continuously at work trying to accommodate themselves to the demands you place upon them. From a struc-tural point of view, muscles aren't very needy organs. Barring disease or trauma and provided with a sufficient amount of nutrients, they will remain healthy for more than a century. However, from a functional point of view, muscles have very specific needs. To permit fluid, flexible, and frictionless movement with the least amount of resistance across the joint as possible, muscles need to be restored to their optimal length daily.

All muscles have a unique optimal muscle length, or O.M.L., which ex-presses itself as the ability to permit the full range of motion at the joint it serves with no restriction. Because they are highly adaptive organs that constantly change their length, muscles often fall short of their O.M.L.—literally. Every position you assume initiates the building of bridges across the myofilaments, causing muscles to shorten. Although changing your position erases many of these bridges, rem-nants remain. These leftovers prevent your muscles from returning to their proper and intended lengths. This means that when you next move, your muscles operate with diminished capacity. These shortened muscles inhibit full movement, ren-dering you less flexible. The less flexible you are, the stiffer your joints and the more limited their range of motion. As a joint's range is reduced, the surface of its carti-lage will not be fully lubricated. This makes the joint far more susceptible to wear and tear and leads to a variety of dysfunctions, not the least of which is degenerative arthritis. In addition, shortness creates an imbalance between antagonistic muscles and their oppositional counterparts. When one muscle is dysfunctional, its complementary muscle has to work harder to compensate for the deficit. In an attempt to restore balance around the joint, the overburdened complementary muscle will shorten. Now you have a situation where both muscles in the pair are working at a deficiency. This imposes pressure on the joint and accelerates its wear and tear. In essence, the whole system is thrown off kilter. And the problems don't end there.

Repetitive movements and prolonging a position's duration leave a greater residue of bridges, which accumulate within the myofilaments. The longer the bridges remain, the stronger they are attached and the more permanently affixed the resulting shortened position becomes. The shorter the muscle, the tighter it is. The tighter a muscle, the more it imposes additional stress on the joint. The more overburdened a joint, the more prone it is to degeneration and injury. This dysfunctional chain of events accounts for the majority of chronic aches and pain. It doesn't matter whether you are an extremely active or relatively sedentary person: Every position you assume initiates the same physiological processes.

To maintain the optimal functional capabilities of skeletal muscles, their O.M.L. needs to be maintained. When you elongate or stretch muscles to their optimal length continuously for 30 seconds, something truly remarkable occurs. There is a special organ that lives within the tendon (see *golgi tendon apparatus*, below) that sends a message to the muscle fibers to let go of the bridges they have built. This effectively wipes the slate clean. By using therapeutic movements to stretch your muscles in a specifically prescribed way daily, you enable them to produce the smooth, balanced, and pain-free movements they were designed to deliver.

Tendons

ANATOMICAL DESCRIPTION If skeletal muscles were attached directly to bone, they would rip under the strain of movement. Nature's solution is to taper skeletal muscles at their ends into fibrous cords of connective tissue called tendons. The tendon fibers extend from the muscle to the bone, where they penetrate the bone's outer layer. Embedded as such, they link or anchor muscles firmly to the bones they serve. When a muscle contracts, the tendon pulls on the bone to cause a movement. By virtue of their enormous strength, tendons enable muscles to produce movement without tearing.

Inside the tendon lives a fascinating organ called the *golgi tendon apparatus,* whose sole function is to protect the tendon and its muscle from damage. It is a receptor that responds to excessive levels of muscle tension by inhibiting further muscle contraction. When movement becomes hazardous, for instance, lifting an extremely heavy object, the golgi send a message to the muscle fibers to let go of the contraction. While movement of the tendon is a voluntary act, the reflex of the golgi is an involuntary response to danger. Without this built-in safeguard, tendons and their muscles would be completely vulnerable to the forces of overexertion.

BIOLOGICAL NEEDS The relationships among the anatomical elements of the musculoskeletal system are so intimate that when you promote the health of your tendons, both the muscles from which they extend and the bones to which they connect benefit. Tendons need to be restored to their optimal length daily for two very important reasons. First, when a tendon is stretched, it pulls on the bone. The body responds to this stimulation by diverting calcium to the source of the increased stress and demand, the tendon and bone. The additional calcium increases the strength of the tendon *and* increases bone production at the site of the attachment. The net effect is that the whole attachment is strengthened. Second, when you engage the tendon in a prolonged stretch of 30 seconds to 1 minute, the golgi tendon apparatus is triggered. Because the golgi perceives the prolonged stretch as overexertion, it responds by sending a signal to the muscle fibers to release the bridges they have built throughout the day. Thus the muscle is able to let go of its shortened position and return to its O.M.L.

The Spine

The ability to stand on two feet and walk erect makes us distinctly human. This posture is made possible by the unique structure and function of the *spine*. The *spinal column* runs right down the middle of the human body, forming its core. It is a strong, flexible structure that holds the head and trunk upright, provides the ideal curvature to withstand the forces of gravity, and houses the nervous system's main informational highway, the *spinal cord*. The spine is made up of 33 *vertebrae*, which are linked to a series of movable *joints*. *Discs,* which act as shock absorbers, are sandwiched between the vertebrae. *Ligaments* and *muscles* complete the picture and give the spine the support and strength it needs to function optimally.

The Spinal Column

ANATOMICAL DESCRIPTION Almost all movement utilizes or affects your spine, and for this reason the spine is the source of the greatest amount of dysfunction. In fact, more people suffer from lower-back pain than any other type of chronic ailment. I left the spinal column for last because it is made up of all the different anatomical elements we've examined thus far, including bones (here, vertebrae), joints, cartilage, ligaments, and muscles. While some new physiological components will be introduced, much of the spine's structure and function will be familiar.

The spinal column is made up of 33 irregular bones (vertebrae) that are stacked one on top of each other, creating a flexible column or chain (see 3–3). There are three main types of movable vertebrae: *cervical,* which are located in the neck and allow the head to move up, down, left, right, and side to side; *thoracic,* which are located in the upper back and form joints with the ribs; and *lumbar,* which are located in the lower back and bear most of the body's weight. In addition, there are two main types of fused vertebrae: the *sacral,* which are located at the base of the spine and connect to the pelvis; and the *coccyx,* which form the tail

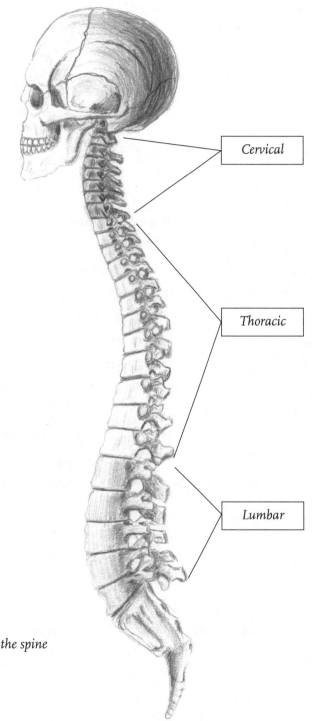

Cervical

Thoracic

Lumbar

3–3. Illustration of the spine

or end tip of the spine; neither has a functional role. The names for these five distinct kinds of vertebrae also refer to the five distinct curved areas that give the spinal column its characteristic shape.

It took nearly 4 million years of trial and error for nature to perfect the unique curvature of the spine. When viewed from the side, it appears as an S. This curve gives the spine its ability to support the body's weight, the capacity to withstand the constant pull of gravity, and the resilience to absorb the impact of constant movement. So perfected is its design that many human-made structures, such as bridges, have been constructed with its engineering blueprint in mind. It provides just the right amount of balance, strength, and flexibility we need to engage with our environment. Without this unique curvature, we would simply be unable to lead the kinds of lives that we do. .

Sandwiched between the vertebrae is another structural splendor of the human body, the spinal *discs*. These tough, pliable discs are made up of two parts: a nucleus (interior) composed of a supple gel-like substance (80 percent water, 20 percent protein) and an annulus (exterior) consisting of more than two thousand layers or concentric rings of connective tissue (see 3–4). The discs provide a natural buffer, protecting the individual vertebrae from rubbing against each other. Even more significantly, they act as shock absorbers for the entire spinal structure. When vertebrae are compressed under the strain of movement and gravity, the disc transfers the pressure to the vertebra directly below it. The disc's malleability permits the forces of compression to be distributed evenly so that no matter what position the body is in, the compressive forces are borne optimally. This ensures that no pressure ever falls more upon one area of a vertebra than another. The discs also permit the smooth and fluid movement of the spine.

Movement of the spine, as in the rest of the body, is made possible through joints. Those located in the spine are called *facet joints,* which are a type of synovial joints. They connect two vertebrae together and facilitate the ability to bend forward, arch backward, lean from side to side, and turn in either direction. The structure and function of facet joints are similar to the synovial joints that we looked at earlier in the chapter. Their makeup includes joint capsules, which pro-

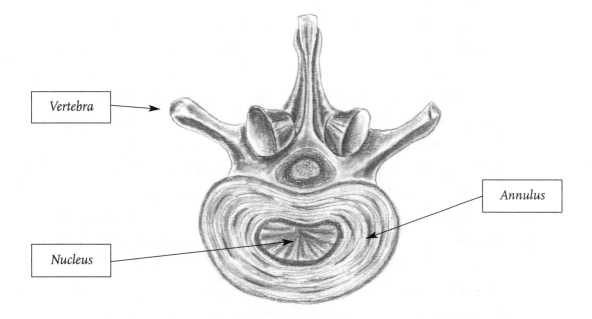

Vertebra

Annulus

Nucleus

3–4. Illustration of a disc

vide nourishment and lubrication; cartilage, which protects their bony ends; ligaments, which support the capsule and hold the vertebrae in place; and muscle,
which move them. Each facet joint allows for only a limited amount of movement,
but taken together, these small movements make the spine very flexible.

BIOLOGICAL NEEDS The spine is the centerpiece of the human structure. All
of the most important anatomical elements are either attached to or housed within
it, and almost all functions involve it in some way. This interconnectedness and in-
terdependency means that the benefits of a well-tuned spine extend to the entire
body. In aiming at optimal musculoskeletal health, the spine is the bull's-eye.

When you treat your back poorly, it treats you back poorly. Active participation in life is utterly impossible when there's dysfunction of the spine. Anyone
who's been there knows what I'm talking about: It takes you out of circulation.
Conversely, active participation in life is effortless when the spine functions well.
Maintaining and sustaining the health of your spine is easy. Once again, movement is the key.

The facet joints of the spine need to be moved through their full range of motion daily so that their cartilage is lubricated and nourished. The muscles that connect and mobilize the facet joints need to be moved to their extreme ends so that their O.M.L. is restored. In this way the spine responds like any other joint-related structure in the body. However, the spine has two additional needs that make it unique: the maintenance of good posture and a certain amount of rest each day. What is the link between these two special requirements? Gravity.

Gravity is the force that keeps our feet on the ground, preventing us from floating off into space. As you read in Chapter 2, there are many professionals in the medical community who maintain that the human body is ill equipped to withstand the forces of gravity. They point to the overwhelming statistics of chronic lower back pain as proof of this. They're pointing their finger in the wrong direction. The problem is not the laws of physics but how we choose to live within the parameters of those laws. In fact NASA, in a series of landmark studies on the effects of weightlessness and astronauts, proved that we're not only biomechanically predisposed for gravity (we even come equipped with antigravitational muscles) but utterly dependent on it for our survival.[2]

Gravity pulls us down toward earth. If you think back to the biological needs of bones, you will see why this is beneficial. When bones are pulled, the allocation of calcium is increased at the source of the stress. The increase in calcium causes bones to become sturdier and stronger. With gravity, there is a constant pulling on all bones. Thus an increased proportion of calcium is diverted equally throughout the skeleton, causing the entire structure to be made sturdier and stronger. It is important to note that in the absence of gravity, bone releases calcium from its storehouse and thins down and degrades. For example, astronauts have been known to lose as much as 200 milligrams of calcium a day in space.[3] However, for gravity to remain beneficial, good posture needs to be maintained so that the forces acting on the structure are distributed appropriately.

Posture or spinal alignment has a direct effect on where the line of gravity falls. Ideally, it should fall directly on our center of gravity. What is our center of gravity? The human body is balanced upon a vertical axis that moves within a three-dimensional space separated by three planes. These planes are the *sagittal plane,* which divides the body into right and left sections; the *frontal plane,* which divides the body into front and back sections; and the *transverse plane,* which divides the body into upper and lower sections. The point at which these planes converge is the center of the human body—right around your navel. This is the center of gravity. Proper spinal alignment forces the line of gravity to be centered (see 3–5, page 70) directly over the base of support at the feet, which allows the joints and muscles responsible for maintaining our posture to do so with the least amount of resistance and energy. I cannot overstate the importance of proper posture for the health of the body. Misalignment or poor posture causes unequal load-bearing and imbalance of the musculature (see 3–6, page 71). Under these disabling conditions, the musculoskeletal system has to overcompensate to keep itself upright. This overcompensation comes at a very high price: Muscles hang or tug on the structure, rather than support it, and joints become overburdened; discs that are designed to function with a normal load of pressure begin to herniate or slip under the excess burden; and vertebrae, left without the additional protection of their cushiony shock absorbers, are riddled with microtraumatic injuries. Dysfunction then is not the fault of gravity but one of our own making. To help gravity help us, we need to stand up straight. For this essential reason, I have included postural therapeutic movements in Chapter 7.

Another benefit of gravity is that it helps to maintain the shape of the S curve of the spine. In fact, the S shape is a direct response to the forces of gravity. After all, the theory of evolution presupposes that the anatomical characteristics that have survived are ones that have bettered our species. The worst traits died out long ago. Regardless, by constantly pulling on the spine, gravitational forces actually enlarge the curve during the day, making it more pronounced. This prevents the spine from becoming too straight and thus unable to bear the burden of movement. However, as the curve deepens, the discs between the vertebrae become thinner. The constant compression squeezes the contents out of them. This is why you are shorter at the end of the day. But remember, the human body works on a give-and-take basis, and a really wonderful thing happens to compensate for

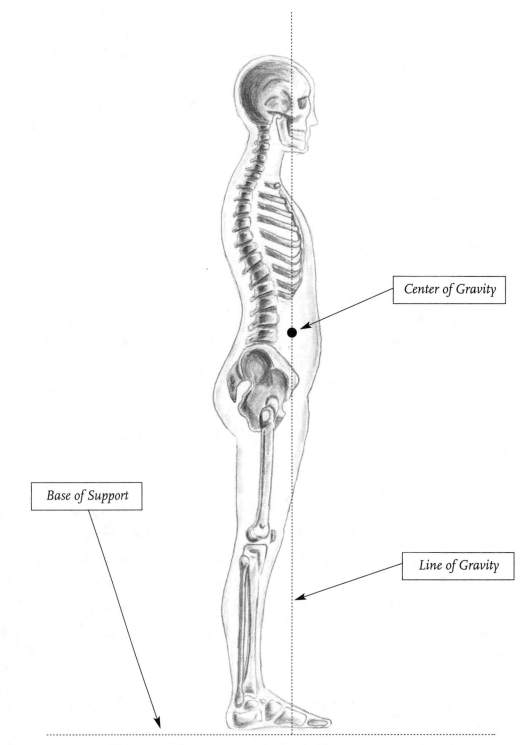

3–5. *Illustration of proper posture in relationship to the center of gravity*

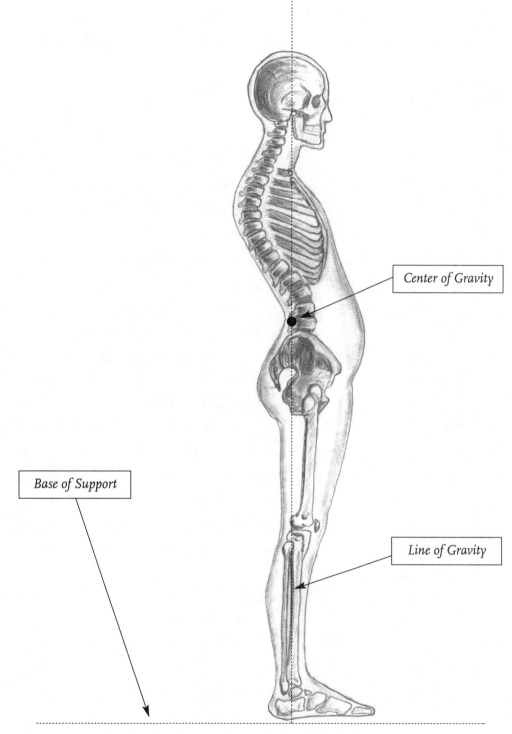

Center of Gravity

Base of Support

Line of Gravity

3–6. Illustration of poor posture in relationship to the center of gravity

the by-products of gravity. The whole system revives itself at night. Sleep provides the spine the time it needs to unload the effects of gravitational forces. The discs refill and resume their natural thickness. All returns to normal, in preparation for a new day to begin.

Use It or Lose It

Musculoskeletal dysfunction is a by-product of neglect. The consequence of this neglect is pain. If you fail to maintain the health of your muscles and joints, they will in return fail you. Likewise, if you are consistent in caring for them, they will reward you in kind. In the final analysis, you've got to use your body and keep it free of dysfunction or you will lose the ability to move it.

Unfortunately, our modern lifestyle doesn't promote the full range of movement that our body requires for optimal health. While our steady progress in science and technology has certainly made living easier, it has also made it harder on the body. Being a sitting culture has left us with a deficiency of movement that extends far beyond the chair. We no longer use our lower extremities to run after prey or run from predators. We no longer use our upper extremities to reach for fruit or climb trees. And we no longer walk long distances over rugged terrain or swim rivers and oceans as a means of travel. Today, if we do attempt activities of this kind or anything remotely similar, it is with muscles and joints that are now completely unprepared and thus vulnerable to injury. In fact, it takes as little as six to eight hours of biomechanical idleness to bring about a reduction in musculoskeletal capacity.

Yet we want to be inactive for prolonged periods of time then jolt our systems with activity. We want to sit around all day then play tennis, jog, go to a yoga class, or dance at night. And we want to do this free of pain. Don't expect evolution to lend a hand. We can't possibly adapt when we're sending our bodies such mixed signals. It seems we can't have it both ways. Or can we?

I am here to tell you that we can. Now some of you might think that I'm going to suggest reverting to a life of squatting, foraging for food, or turning back the clock in some other fashion. As promised in my introduction to this book, I will not ask you to make any changes to your lifestyle. What I am going to do is provide you with a program that supplements your deficiency of movement. As you have just seen, the problems associated with the anatomical elements involved in movement are highly complex. Yet the solution for maintaining their care is simple. However, there is a great deal of precision needed to move them in just the right way to achieve optimal musculoskeletal health. Every joint in the body has a unique prescribed range of motion, and every muscle has a specific O.M.L. It is an exact science. The good news is that Part II of this book eliminates *all* the guesswork for you. I have spent my life honing and solidifying the Weisberg Way. My therapeutic movements are designed with the utmost accuracy to restore your muscles to their proper length and to take your joints through their full range of possible motion. The result of doing my program daily will be a pain-free life.

Happy Endings: Christy's Story

Christy S., age 25, is a spirited and energetic stay-at-home mom with two children. Her story illustrates the devastating effects of a deficiency of movement. After being immobile for more than four months, she engaged in some ordinary and innocuous activity that left her with a sprained hip, strained muscles, and severe piriformis syndrome.

I now understand why Dr. Weisberg's motto is: "Life is movement and movement is life." Although I have always been an active person, I never fully realized how fundamentally important movement was until I suffered the consequences of not moving.

When I was pregnant with my first child, I was diagnosed with a condition that required bed rest for the duration of my pregnancy. This was very difficult for me because I was a very athletic person. Given the situation, however, I proceeded to spend four months almost completely motionless. When I was more than halfway through my pregnancy, my doctor told me that I didn't have the condition after all and that my activity levels could return to normal. One morning shortly after, I was making my bed when I felt a terrible pain in my groin. Because I had played sports throughout my life, I thought I had pulled a muscle there. Although I couldn't imagine how I had injured myself tucking in a bedsheet, I treated it as such by immediately icing and wrapping it. However, after a few weeks my pain was getting more severe. I started taking 800 to 1,000 mg of ibuprofen a day to see if that would help, but still my pain would not go away. I went to my primary care doctor, but his tests, including X-rays and MRIs, yielded nothing conclusive. After a few months, I became really concerned. I always thought that as you got older a certain amount of deterioration would make it harder to bounce back, but I was young and unable to recover. It didn't make sense to me. As the pain got worse, I started doing less and less, which seemed to increase my pain more and more. It got so debilitating that I ended up back in bed.

I was feeling utterly hopeless. Then my mother referred me to Dr. Weisberg. He told me that my injury was a consequence of immobility and explained that immobility weakens the musculature in the body to such a degree that it leaves both muscles and joints vulnerable when doing the simplest of tasks. It takes only six weeks of immobility for muscular strength to be reduced by *half.* Because I was in bed for triple that amount of time, my muscles were too weak to work properly. Under these conditions, the minute I started using my body in any capacity, I was at risk for injury.

The first thing Dr. Weisberg did was to get me moving appropriately again. Because I was still pregnant, we had to proceed slowly. Within a few weeks of doing his targeted therapeutic movement, I felt relief. Then he showed me the 3-Minute Maintenance Method, which I added to my daily routine. By the time I gave birth, I was completely pain free. I have remained that way for one reason: I rarely miss a day of the Weisberg Way. I learned from my experience that being sedentary weakens the body in the same way that immobility does. I also learned that even a person as active as I am can't possibly target all muscle groups and joints adequately every day. I like to think of the program as a vitamin (and it's an easy pill to swallow) that I take to supplement any movement deficiencies that my muscles or joints may have so that they are preserved for a lifetime.

4: Medicinal Know-No's

YOU'RE IN PAIN. Your lower back is out, and your knees ache. Maybe you have a splitting headache, and your neck is stiff. Or perhaps your shoulder hurts, and your arthritic hands are sore. Whatever its source, the pain is preventing you from moving forward with your day. You want it to stop, and you want it to stop fast. What do you do? If you're like millions of other people around the world, your first course of action is to pop a pill. What happens after you take it? Most likely, within 20 minutes your pain will have disappeared. It works! You go about your business and life returns to normal. Problem solved? Well, not exactly.

Drugs are supposed to do for the human body what it can't do for itself. For the most part, the human body needs very little assistance. That's because it is a healing machine. Left to its own biochemical devices, it has the capacity to reverse infections, repair physiological structures, and restore function to internal organs. In the absence of intervention, the human body can withstand and prevail over sickness and infirmity. However, it can also capitulate and succumb to them. Because of this, humankind has, for thousands of years, looked for ways to assist and enhance the natural mechanisms that promote well-being. Eastern cultures pioneered the use of herbs and botanicals to stimulate and improve the physiological immune processes. Western culture focused on crisis intervention with an emphasis on medicines that inhibit or supplant the body's immunological processes.

Although medicinal intervention has vastly improved our all-around level of health care, it comes at a price.

Every time you introduce a drug into your body, there are both benefits and drawbacks. Taking medication is always a compromise: Medication interferes with the body's finely tuned regulatory systems that are responsible for healing. There are times when a drug's therapeutic or curative advantage far outweighs any corresponding disadvantages. For instance, when the body is incapable of healing itself, as with many diseases, drugs help to thwart, eliminate, and even regress the pathology. In these instances a drug's shortcomings pale in comparison with its lifesaving abilities.

However, there are times when a drug is more of a liability than an asset. For instance, some medications have little or no therapeutic value but are taken either to speed up the immune response or mask the symptoms of an underlying cause. When the body is capable of healing itself by its own restorative powers, medication can lessen its ability to manage the crisis on its own. This often contributes to the perpetuation of the primary condition. Such is the case with chronic musculoskeletal dysfunction.

Musculoskeletal dysfunction expresses itself in a variety of ways. The most frequently occurring symptoms are inflamed swollen joints, tight spasmodic muscles, and recurrent chronic pain. In an otherwise healthy person, these symptoms are indications that the body is responding and coping appropriately. I know it's hard to fathom that such uncomfortable, even if not debilitating, symptoms are a normal and necessary part of the healing process, but each symptom in its own way is exactly that. In fact, symptoms are a protective response to an injury. The more severe the injury, the greater the response and thus the

Pain and inflammation are signs that a healthy healing process is underway.

greater the repair. Nonetheless, these symptoms can be bothersome and often interfere with the regular function of your daily life. It isn't hard to see why you'd want to make them go away as soon as they arise.

There is a veritable smorgasbord of manufactured medicines, herbs, and other medicinal compounds that target the symptoms associated with musculoskeletal dysfunction. They come in a multitude of shapes, sizes, and brands. Some are swallowed while others are placed under your tongue. Some are worn as patches while others are injected into your bloodstream. You can even grow some in your backyard. Regardless of how these remedies are packaged, they generally fall into one of three classes: *anti-inflammatories, muscle relaxants,* and *analgesics.* All these medications reduce or eliminate the symptoms of musculoskeletal dysfunction. That's why millions of people have come to depend upon them. In fact,

- Close to 200 million people regularly take over-the-counter or prescription medications for the symptoms of musculoskeletal dysfunction.[1]

- Fifty percent of chronic pain sufferers take from one to five medications a day (of them, 25 percent will abuse or become addicted to their medications).[2]

- Approximately $6.6 billion is spent annually on pain medications.[3]

Although drugs are highly effective at relieving symptoms, their effects are only temporary. Once they wear off, symptoms usually return. What do you do then? You take more drugs. But once again, symptoms return. So begins the self-perpetuating, viscious pain-relief cycle. Though the medications certainly make you feel better initially, they are unable to actually make you better. To date, there are no magic pills or potions, teas or tonics that can actually *cure* musculoskeletal dysfunction. Though some, including, in particular, herbs and nutritional supplements, can enhance muscular rejuvenation, bone production, and cartilage regeneration, none can bring about lasting improvement. In other words, you get relief without resolution. And *feeling* well without *being* well is a slippery slope. Because drugs mask the indications of dysfunction, the dysfunction is allowed to progress unchecked. The longer it remains unresolved, the more exacerbated it becomes. As the condition worsens, so too will its corresponding symptoms. As they become increasingly un-

The Tortoise and the Hare: In our fast-paced, fast-food society, we expect fast relief. Although therapeutic movements may take longer than drugs, they produce more permanent relief. Remember that a slow and steady healing process always wins the race.

bearable, more potent drugs are then often relied on to make them go away. In fact, with or without drugs, symptoms will continue until the underlying cause is addressed.

There is only one cure for musculoskeletal dysfunction: therapeutic movements. My therapeutic movements (see Chapter 7) bring about biomechanical repair by stimulating the biochemical and physiological processes responsible for healing. And they do so at a pace to which your body can easily adapt and thereby produce real change. This is a deliberate and methodical process that takes from two to six weeks of consistent application to eradicate most dysfunction. Although drugs may be faster at relieving symptoms, they often slow down the healing process. That's because drugs alter the body's biochemical landscape, thus reducing the effectiveness of naturally occurring response systems.

Given these facts, you may be wondering why so many doctors encourage the use of a variety of pain medications. The medical community defines chronic pain by its duration. Any pain that persists for more than six months is often seen as a manifestation of a malfunctioning pain-response system. Likewise, chronic inflammation and recurrent muscle spasms are often seen as by-products of systems that have somehow gone berserk. In other words, they are not perceived as symptoms of a problem but as problems in and of themselves. While there are instances where this is true, they are, by far, in the minority. To combat these misperceived abnormalities, doctors usually turn to their most tried and true weapon: medication. Because drugs quickly bring about relief, the treatment is considered a success. But once again the underlying biomechanical condition is left unresolved.

Are there ever times when taking drugs for musculoskeletal pain is appropriate? Of course there are. I want to provide you with all the essential information you'll need to make informed choices in the face of symptoms. I want you to have the ability to weigh a drug's benefits and drawbacks so that you become an active participant in your own treatment. And I want you to think a little bit before popping your next pill. It amazes me that while hundreds of millions of people take pain medications almost every day of their lives, very few of them know what the drugs do, how they do it, or what their risks and side effects are. What follows is a guide to the drugs taken for relieving the symptoms of chronic pain. I will explore all three classes of drugs mentioned earlier in the chapter, starting with the most used and accessible, over-the-counter anti-inflammatories, and ending with the least used and accessible, prescription narcotic analgesics. Finally, I will conclude with an in-depth look at alternative therapies, including herbs and botanicals and food and nutritional supplements. Being able to know when to say no and when to say yes will go a long way in maintaining your optimal health. However, before taking any medication you should first work through my 7 Steps to Immediate Relief (see page 153) to alleviate pain, inflammation, stiffness, muscle spasm, and other manifestations of biomechanical dysfunction.

Nonsteroidal Anti-Inflammatory Drugs (NSAIDs)

MOST COMMONLY TAKEN Many NSAIDs, including aspirin (Bayer, Bufferin), ibuprofen (Advil, Motrin), and naproxen (Aleve, Naprosyn), are available over the counter. Stronger NSAIDs, including Anaprox, Celebrex, and Bextra, require a prescription from your doctor.

MEDICINAL KNOW-NO'S There are some very good reasons why hundreds of millions of people around the world take NSAIDs for pain regularly. They are easily obtained, inexpensive, and convenient to carry. Most important, they get the job done and get it done fast. NSAIDs are highly effective at relieving a wide spectrum of symptomatic aches and pains. Everything, from shin splints to throbbing headaches, dissipates within a half-hour of intake. So what's the harm in a little relief? A lot, as it turns out.

NSAIDs stop pain by blocking proinflammatory prostaglandins, hormones responsible for causing inflammation. Because inflammation produces pain, reducing the mechanism that causes inflammation reduces the pain. But is this a good thing? Inflammation is a healthy manifestation of the body's immune system. It is a natural, essential, and well-regulated response to an area's being injured in some way. The process of inflammation begins when a macrotraumatic or, in musculoskeletal dysfunction, microtraumatic event occurs. Proinflammatory prostaglandins cause a dilation of blood vessels, which allows for an increased flow of blood to the damaged area. The enhanced circulation brings about an increase in the amount of healing nutrients and immune cells that work to rectify the underlying problem. The presence of additional fluids will cause uncomfortable swelling, but this is only a by-product of the injury's bringing about its own recovery. Allowed to run its course and tempered by naturally occurring anti-inflammatory prostaglandins, the injury heals and the inflammation subsides. Thus the inflammatory process makes recovery happen faster. On the other hand, NSAIDs slow down and interfere with this process. Even when they cause a temporary abatement of symptoms, the dysfunction remains. In fact, the loss of immunization agents to the area results in a prolonging and worsening of the injury. That is why, as so often happens, when the medication wears off, the pain returns.

Did You Know That . . .

- **More than 30 million people take NSAIDs every day?**[4]
- **Each year in the United States alone more than 103,000 people are hospitalized from the serious side effects of NSAIDs?**[5]
- **Of those people more than 16,500 die?**[6]

NSAIDs also stop pain when there is no inflammation present. While it isn't entirely clear how this happens, one theory suggests that they block nerve receptors in the injured area, thus making it less receptive to pain. Once again, is this a good thing? The human body comes equipped with pain receptors for the specific purpose of preventing one from using an injured area until the healing process is complete. NSAIDs allow for the opposite to occur. By eliminating the pain, they enable you to resume activities. But this does you a great disservice. Without pain as your guide, you simply cannot calculate the effect that these activities have on your injury. Chances are that you are doing the very things that to heal you shouldn't be doing. The net effect is that the problem is compounded and the injury is perpetuated indefinitely until proper treatment is administered to the underlying cause.

SIDE EFFECTS NSAIDs have serious side effects, some of which can result in death. Most severe is their adverse effect on the stomach. While going about the business of blocking the biochemistry responsible for pain and inflammation, NSAIDs also block enzymes responsible for generating the mucus that lines and protects the stomach. The consequences of this are bleeding, ulcers, and, if the penetration is near an artery, unstoppable hemorrhaging. To combat this, drug companies released a new class of NSAIDs called COX-2 inhibitors, of which Celebrex and Bextra are the best known. These NSAIDs have less impact on the stomach-protecting enzymes and reduce gastrointestinal side effects by almost 50 percent. Unfortunately, COX-2 inhibitors can triple the risk of heart attacks.[7] Moreover these new NSAIDs cost around 4,000 percent more per pill than their older counterparts, yet relieve pain no better. In addition, they have side effects, such as diarrhea and sinus irritation, and are a risk to people with high blood pressure and bleeding problems.

Taking NSAIDs occasionally and *as directed* will not likely cause any significant, irreparable, or fatal damage. However, they are not only the most used, they are also among the most abused medications in the world. Prolonged dependence coupled with exceeding the normal dosage will put you at risk for serious side effects.

Generally perceived as innocuous and benign, NSAIDs are in fact highly potent drugs. Their easy availability certainly adds to this misperception, but the fault is with the takers, not the makers. Therefore, if you find yourself in a situation that calls for their ingestion, you should take them judiciously, pragmatically, and on an extremely limited basis.

WHEN TO SAY YES *If used properly,* NSAIDs can have considerable medicinal value. For instance, it is highly appropriate to take NSAIDs any time nonmechanical bodily pain is excruciating and unbearable, such as from toothaches, menstrual cramps, and urinary tract infections. Likewise, NSAIDs are suitable when musculoskeletal pain reaches an intolerable level and prohibits you from using therapeutic movements for healing. NSAIDs are highly effective at eradicating symptoms without promoting the dependence and buildup of tolerance that narcotics do.

In addition, NSAIDs reduce prolonged exposure to inflammation. An extended influx of nutrients can break down damaged tissue rather than build it up. The key here is being able to distinguish at what point the healing process has gone from helpful to harmful. The telltale signs are when the painful area is warm and swollen and if the swelling has lasted for more than two weeks. When these symptoms are present, NSAIDs can be highly beneficial. However, they should be used only as a last resort, not as the initial or only treatment. Remember that when you are taking medication, use of the injured or painful area should be kept to an absolute minimum.

Steroidal Anti-Inflammatory Drugs (Corticosteroids)

MOST COMMONLY TAKEN When you hear the word "steroid," it may conjure up the image of weight lifters or athletes who take them to produce exceedingly large muscles. However, there are actually many different classes of steroids, some of which are used to treat inflammation and pain. Corticosteroids, which include Cortone, Decadron, and Prednisone, are dispensed only by prescription.

MEDICINAL KNOW-NO'S Corticosteroids are very potent drugs that are used for a wide variety of disorders that include allergies and cancer. From a musculoskeletal standpoint, prescription of these drugs is usually reserved for disease-related symptoms, such as the pain associated with rheumatoid arthritis, because of the long list of serious side effects that accompany their intake. However, many doctors do prescribe them for severe flare-ups of acute mechanical dysfunction. Although they fall under the anti-inflammatory umbrella, corticosteroids bare little resemblance to their nonsteroidal counterparts, which we just discussed. In fact, their modality is so complex that a complete understanding of how they work was only recently arrived at. What we now know about corticosteroids paints a discomforting picture.

Corticosteroids are produced naturally in the body. They are powerful anti-inflammatory hormones that act to counterbalance the proinflammatory prostaglandin hormone. When an injury occurs, proinflammatory prostaglandins cause the area to become inflamed. The buildup of fluids enhances the healing process by eliminating toxins, repairing tissue, and flooding the site of the injury with essential restorative cells. At the same time, the adrenal cortex releases corticosteroids into the bloodstream, where they inhibit proinflammatory prostaglandin production. The amount of steroids released depends on how much the body needs to moderate between the two hormones. When it comes to the complex interplay of biochemistry, this natural, self-regulating system gives you just the right amount of what you need when you need it.

Corticosteroids are also produced synthetically. They can be introduced into the body orally or by injection. Either way, they are variant reproductions of their naturally occurring counterpart and act to mimic the way they reduce inflammation, albeit at an accelerated pace. Herein lies the problem. Synthetic corticosteroids can cause a rapid reduction of inflammation, but they do so at the expense of the slower-acting immunization properties. Thus they upset the delicate balance between proinflammatory prostaglandins and natural corticosteroids. Furthermore, the presence of synthetic corticosteroids usurps the function of the adrenal cortex,

Did You Know That . . .

▪ **Arthritis sufferers who take steroidal or nonsteroidal anti-inflammatory medications incur worse damage to their joints than people who take nothing?**[8]

▪ **There is a long list of serious side effects associated with the use of steroids yet they are still widely prescribed?**

▪ **Steroids should be taken only in the most severe cases?**

which responds by shutting down. Within six weeks of this forced prolonged inactivity, it can begin to atrophy. Because the adrenal cortex plays a complex role in many biological systems, including blood coagulation and the immune response to infection, when it ceases to play its intended role, those systems with which it is involved are left vulnerable to many problems.

To avoid these and other catastrophic side effects, doctors usually prescribe corticosteroids for only short periods of time—usually 7 to 10 days—unless the problem extends into the realm of disease. They are drugs that should not be administered lightly and should always be taken with the utmost consideration and caution.

SIDE EFFECTS Synthetic corticosteroids trigger a series of highly invasive and complex biochemical reactions that, from their initial ingestion, affects a surprising variety of different biological systems. The most severe of these is the compromise to the immune system. By suppressing the immunization process, corticosteroids mask the various symptoms of infection. Depending on the severity of the infection, the situation can easily progress from dangerous to life threatening. Less imposing but no less serious side effects from intake for a short term are gastrointestinal upset, nausea, dizziness, and headaches. If any of these persist, you should contact your doctor immediately.

The side effects from long-term intake—more than 7 to 10 days—include extreme bloating and water retention, thin and brittle bones, muscle weakness and loss of muscle mass, adrenal and pituitary gland suppression, black-and-blue marks, convulsions, ulcers, potassium loss, insomnia, weight gain, mood swings, and blood clots. In addition, long-term use may significantly increase the risk of cataracts and glaucoma, heart failure, high blood pressure, diabetes, and osteoporosis. And this is just a partial list. It is imperative that these drugs be carefully considered and used only under careful supervision.

WHEN TO SAY YES The long list of dangerous side effects makes it difficult to be an advocate of corticosteroids. However, there are times when they can be highly effective at making one's life more manageable. For instance, corticosteroids can be very beneficial to people suffering from disease or trauma-related inflammation. In these instances, the body continues to try to repair an area that cannot be repaired. It simply will not give up trying to heal itself. Thus the inflammation mechanism gets stuck on the On switch and itself becomes a chronic and disabling situation. For nondisease musculoskeletal biomechanical dysfunction, corticosteroids should be only used when the area is unresponsive to all other treatments or in extreme cases of overwhelming inflammation. Even then, they should be given only as a last resort and for a very short time.

Muscle Relaxants

MOST COMMONLY TAKEN There are two types of muscle relaxants, both available only by prescription. Direct muscle relaxers, which include benzodiazepines (Valium, Xanax), work by relaxing the muscle tissue itself. Indirect muscle relaxers, which include Flexeril, Norflex, and Soma, work by sedating the entire body.

MEDICINAL KNOW-NO'S As human beings, we sustain tissue damage and varying degrees of injury daily. We bump into things, trip, fall, cut ourselves, get into awkward positions, and make sudden jolting movements. All these events have an effect on the musculoskeletal system. This is why everyone will, at some point in his or her life, experience a muscle spasm. When the body is in some form of danger, be it from the buildup of microtraumas or a full-blown macrotraumatic event, a muscle spasm acts much like an alert-and-response team. The pain it brings on alerts you to the danger, and the involuntarily contraction of the muscles around the site of injury is its response. This protective spasm allows the damaged area the time it needs to heal by minimizing movement, function, and continued irritation. Most muscle spasms tend to go away in a short period of time. Stretching, massaging, or getting up and moving around usually alleviates them immediately; however, some last longer. The longer a spasm lasts, the greater the underlying dysfunction that caused it to occur. When muscle spasms persist, medications are often prescribed.

Muscle relaxants stop spasms by relaxing muscles. How do they do it? The brain sends neural impulses to the muscles by the central nervous system either to activate or inhibit movement. During a spasm, the brain is constantly activating the muscle, which causes severe pain. Direct muscle relaxants go to the source of this activity, the central nervous system. As they prevent intraneural communication between the brain and the muscle, the stimulation for contraction subsides, and so does the spasm. At the same time, direct muscle relaxants increase the neurotransmission of gamma-aminobatyric acid (GABA), which functions to inhibit pain. Indirect muscle relaxants work by suppressing and sedating the entire central nervous system. Because the neural pathways are inhibited, the entire body, including but not limited to muscles, becomes completely relaxed. The more relaxed your body, the more the muscles loosen up and release their contractions. The spasms and the pain subside. No spasm, no pain, no problem, right? Wrong.

First, muscle relaxants are highly addictive. Benzodiazepines in particular are some of the easiest drugs to become hooked on and some of the hardest to kick. Though dependency does not happen overnight, it can occur within a few weeks of continued dosage. Second, muscle relaxants treat the effect of the spasm but not the cause. Without dealing with the cause, the spasm or some other manifestation of dysfunction will surely return. Finally, and perhaps most important for short-term intake, by artificially eliminating the spasm, the body is left without protection. By masking the symptoms of dysfunction you get a false sense of well-being. In fact, muscle relaxants are so potent that you feel as if you have returned to normal a short time after taking them. Without even knowing or feeling it, you begin to incur injury on top of injury, and the dysfunction perpetuates itself. This is why muscle relaxants are another piece of the puzzle in the vicious cycle of chronic pain.

Did You Know That . . .

■ **Muscle relaxants are among the most used and abused medications?**[9]

■ **Muscle relaxants can be more addictive than heroin?**[10]

■ **From 1992 to 1999, emergency room visits for Xanax-related side effects jumped from 16,500 a year to 20,500?**[11]

SIDE EFFECTS Muscle relaxants, especially the direct variety, are among the most abused drugs because they produce feelings of relaxation, sedation, and euphoria. The consequence of this is one of their main side effects: addiction. Although physical dependence does not usually occur with short-term intake (7 to 10 days), it can happen right away for some people.[12] It is therefore important to be aware of your own propensity for addictive or compulsive behavior and proceed accordingly. Once real physical addiction occurs, you must be tapered off the drugs slowly under medical supervision, because the withdrawal symptoms can be very severe and dangerous.

The remaining side effects of muscle relaxants for both short-term and long-term intake are fairly benign. They can induce drowsiness, so it is always important not to operate machinery or drive a car when taking these drugs. They can also cause dizziness, slurred speech, listlessness, and nausea. If any of these symptoms arise, you should consult your doctor immediately.

WHEN TO SAY YES Muscle relaxants are highly appropriate for people suffering from muscular disease. In fact, direct relaxants are one of the drugs of choice for people with multiple sclerosis (MS). They are also extremely useful for stopping the intense spasms associated with a traumatic event. For instance, broken bones often induce severe contractions in their attached muscles. The high intensity can pull the bones farther apart and make them impossible to set. Stopping the spasm with medication is mandatory in this instance. Nondisease-related or trauma-related mechanical dysfunction, such as severe sprains (torn ligaments) and severe strains (torn muscles), can also bring about highly intense spasms. These powerful overcontractions can pull joints out of position and cause them to dislocate. Here, too, muscle relaxants are very appropriate.

Likewise, when the pain from less severe biomechanically induced spasms is overwhelming and persistent, these medications can be beneficial, especially if taken while simultaneously treating the cause. In these instances I recommend taking them at night, as the likelihood of reinjury is very low during sleep.

Nonnarcotic Analgesics: Acetaminophen

MOST COMMONLY TAKEN Acetaminophen is an over-the-counter analgesic or painkiller. By far the most widely used and recognized brand is Tylenol. Others include Aspirin Free Anacin and Apacet.

MEDICINAL KNOW-NO'S Acetaminophen is a safe painkilling agent that produces few side effects. Unlike many prescription analgesics, acetaminophen contains no narcotics. While this reduces its painkilling effect, the resulting risks are reduced as well. And unlike other OTCs, such as NSAIDs, acetaminophen does not have anti-inflammatory properties and so does not interfere with prostaglandin production. However, while acetaminophen doesn't inhibit the naturally occurring immunological process, it also doesn't reduce the inflammation closely tied to musculoskeletal dysfunction. Acetaminophen is purely analgesic: it works by reducing neural impulses along the central nervous system's pathway, thus blocking the perception of pain in the brain. All good—but there is a drawback.

As I've said, pain plays a vital role in the healing process. Not only does it alert you that something is wrong but it helps to produce an appropriate reaction and response. With a macrotraumatic injury, such as breaking a bone, the response is usually quite obvious. But to the imperceptible nature of musculoskeletal microtraumatic injury, the response is less clear. The only reliable indicator that something is amiss is your ability to feel the pain associated with the problem. Acetaminophen shuts down this intraneural communication. By doing so, it inhibits your ability to react and respond in a way that will best facilitate recovery.

Did You Know That . . .

- **More than 175 million American adults take over-the-counter (OTC) medications for pain relief.**[13]
- **58 million of them regularly take Tylenol (acetaminophen).**[14]
- **One-third of adults who use OTCs take more than the recommended dosage.**[15]

SIDE EFFECTS If taken in recommended doses for a short time (7 to 10 days), acetaminophen is practically nontoxic. Excessive or long-term use may cause liver damage, lowered blood-sugar levels, and a yellowing of the skin or the whites of the eyes. Its record of safety and effectiveness has made it the analgesic drug of choice for many medical professionals and has contributed to its overwhelming popularity among patients.

WHEN TO SAY YES When pain goes from being instructive to intrusive, acetaminophen is, bar none, the least invasive way to medicinally subdue it. However, acetaminophen provides only temporary relief and leaves the underlying cause unresolved. If you choose to use it for pain relief, avoid using the injured area and proceed with therapeutic movements as soon as the pain has subsided.

Narcotic Analgesics: Opiates

MOST COMMONLY TAKEN Narcotics are opiate-based analgesics, or painkilling agents, that come in two varieties: short-acting and long-acting. Short-acting narcotics, which include Darvon, Percodan, and Vicodin, produce their painkilling effects quickly and wear off quickly, usually in three to four hours. Long-acting narcotics, which include Methadone, MS Contin, and OxyContin, produce their painkilling effects slowly and wear off slowly, usually after 12 hours.

MEDICINAL KNOW-NO'S Nothing stops pain like narcotics. Simply put, there is less unnecessary pain and suffering in the world because of the job they do. Narcotics are able to relieve much physical misery for people with disease-related pain, such as the pain associated with cancer; they make postoperative surgery and severe trauma more bearable and manageable; and, for some catastrophic pathologies of the nervous system, they can help to make life worth living. However, because of their potency, narcotics should be reserved for these types of extreme cases, *where the pain serves no purpose.* But what about when it does?

Pain from musculoskeletal dysfunction serves a specific purpose and plays a fundamental role in the healing process. The ramification of artificially masking the pain with narcotics, as with many of the other drugs we've explored, is a perpetuation of the dysfunction and the pain. As if this weren't insidious enough, narcotics cause additional problems that need to be considered.

Did You Know That . . .

■ **Approximately 10 million Americans currently use narcotics for chronic pain?**[16]

■ **Americans spent $1.8 billion on narcotic pain medications in the past five years?**[17]

■ **In the past 10 years, annual emergency room visits for narcotic ingestion have more than doubled?**[18]

The human body comes equipped with its own naturally occurring painkilling agents, called endorphins. Endorphins work by blocking nerve receptors in the brain and spinal column. They don't actually deaden the pain; rather, they dissociate you from it. Narcotics are chemically and functionally similar to endorphins. They are a synthetic version derived from the poppy plant, and work in the same way by inhibiting pain impulses sent from nerve receptor sites to the brain. When the body's natural ability to manage pain somehow falls short, narcotics are prescribed as a viable substitute. The problem is that narcotics inhibit the need for endorphin production. The fewer endorphins produced by your body, the more you need painkilling agents from the drug. The more you need from the drug, the higher the dosage needs to be. The higher the dosage, the further the production of endorphins is reduced. And on and on it goes. This process is called the *buildup of tolerance,* and it can occur within *two weeks* of initial intake. With continued use, the body eventually adapts to the drug's presence, and physical dependency occurs. At this point you're not taking the drug just to stop musculoskeletal pain but also to avoid the painful side effects of withdrawal. And if the underlying dysfunction remains unresolved, it will progress along with the physical addiction. Can this cycle ever be broken?

A good way to avoid dependency is by not taking the first pill. Chronic pain is *not* a disease that needs to be treated with drugs. The dysfunction that caused the pain needs to be treated with movement. When you embrace this physiological and biomechanical reality, you will be on the road to a pain-free and drug-free life.

SIDE EFFECTS A very disturbing side effect of narcotics is physical or mental dependency. It is estimated that between 6 and 9 million Americans abuse or are addicted to their pain medications.[19] This is a shocking figure. Sadly, it's not surprising. The past 20 years has seen an enormous increase in the number of people suffering from chronic pain. With little in the way of alternative solutions coupled with the public's desire for a quick fix to its health problems, is it any wonder that we've seen a corresponding increase in the number of prescription drug users? While there is a clear line between use and abuse, it becomes blurred with prolonged intake. Does everyone who takes narcotics become an addict? Of course not. But the harsh truth is that everyone who takes them *can* become an addict. I do believe that addiction to prescription painkillers for legitimate users is unintended. However, as the number of addicts is in the millions, the problem has grown too big to simply be ignored.

On the other hand, I do not want to stigmatize narcotics or scare people away from taking medications that may be their only means of returning to a productive life. Narcotics are a viable source of relief for some, but it would be negligent to disregard that they are also the source of untold problems for others. And while addiction is one of the main side effects of narcotic intake, it isn't the only drawback. Other side effects include nausea and vomiting, dizziness, disorientation, breathing difficulties, uncoordinated muscle movement, minor hallucinations, constipation, depression, and rapid heartbeat. People with disorders in the liver and kidneys must be extra cautious because most narcotics are metabolized in these organs. In the final analysis, the most important determinant factor for use should be the careful assessment of the very real benefits measured against the very real drawbacks.

WHEN TO SAY YES My deep skepticism and critique of narcotics is generally directed at their prescription for the pain from chronic musculoskeletal dysfunction. But even under these circumstances, there are appropriate times to use them. Taken for a short time, narcotics can be enormously helpful in eradicating extreme, unrelenting pain where even a minimal amount of function is impossible. I have also had many patients whose underlying dysfunction had become so severe that the only way to approach rehabilitation was to first break the symptomatic cycle of pain. Once some function was restored, we were able to concentrate on eliminating the root cause of their suffering.

While narcotics shouldn't be the first or only solution of choice, they can get you through a sudden and intensely painful musculoskeletal flare-up. If you do choose to use narcotics, remember that even when the drugs ease your symptoms, the reason you are in pain remains. You must rectify the source of your pain, or you will surely need to be taking narcotics over and over again.

Herbs and Botanicals

MOST COMMONLY TAKEN There are literally thousands of herbs and botanicals used to treat the musculoskeletal system. Some of the more frequently used include bromelain and feverfew (anti-inflammatories), chamomile and kava (muscle relaxants), and boswella and willow bark (analgesics).

MEDICINAL KNOW-NO'S On one hand, herbs and botanicals are perceived as harmless little shrubs and wildflowers that have little or no curative value. Some wonder, "What good can possibly come from celery seeds?" On the other hand, herbs and botanicals are perceived as harmful pills, potions, and powders that are unsound and potentially lethal (and names such as "devil's claw" do not help this image). Still others see herbs and botanicals as a panacea for all the world's illnesses. Don't get an herbalist started on the wonders of horse chestnuts. So which is it? Are herbs and botanicals mundane, menacing, or miraculous? While there's a little bit of truth to all three, don't let the cynicism, names, or hype fool you. Herbs and botanicals should be seen for what they really are: effective yet enigmatic medicines.

The leaves, stems, roots, barks, flowers, and berries of a vast array of herbs and botanicals have been used medicinally for close to 200,000 years. While there is a perception this is mainly a phenomenon of the East, herbs and botanicals have been used in all cultures, by all people, throughout all of history. In fact, herbal medicine, or phytotherapy, is the basis of Western medicine. Though the West veered away from purely herbal remedies (beginning in earnest during the 19th century), approximately 25 percent of all prescription drugs today are derived from herbs and botanicals. Of the remaining 75 percent, some are made from plant extracts while others synthetically mimic their natural counterparts. Given that, you might wonder what exactly is the difference between the two?

Let me start with the similarities. Herbs and botanicals and manufactured medicines are drugs. Both contain bioactive chemicals and compounds that alter numerous processes in the body. Both can produce extremely beneficial results; both can be equally dangerous: just because

Did You Know That . . .

■ **Approximately 130,000 people die each year from prescription pharmaceuticals while fewer than 100 die from consuming herbs?[20]**

■ **23 million Americans use herbal remedies instead of taking prescription medications?[21]**

■ **119 prescription drugs are derived from plants of which 74 percent are used for the same purposes as ancient cultures have used them for thousands of years?[22]**

something is natural doesn't make it less powerful. Therefore, both should be taken with extreme caution and under the direct supervision of a trained practitioner.

This is where the similarities end. Herbs and botanicals are less concentrated than manufactured medications, making them far less potent per dose. Herbs and botanicals produce fewer side effects than most medications and, in stark contrast, are rarely lethal. Herbs and botanicals also contain additional ingredients that seem to interact synergistically with the whole body, whereas medications include only those ingredients designed to target a specific area or problem.

On the other hand, manufactured medicines ensure a consistent amount and specific type of drug per pill while herbal potency and content can vary from plant to plant. Medications are put through rigorous testing before they are made available for public consumption, while only 5,000 of the 500,000 known medicinal herbs and botanicals have been tested in this country so far. The pharmaceutical industry is well regulated, ensuring correct quantity, quality, and safety control; the herbal industry is subjected to absolutely no standards at all. And, for better or worse, manufactured medications relieve symptoms faster than their herbal and botanical counterparts.

The most important consideration for our purposes in comparing herbs and botanicals with manufactured medications is the fundamentally different ways in which they effect the musculoskeletal system. Many herbs and botanicals have anti-inflammatory, antispasmodic, and analgesic properties. While manufactured medicines work by directly supplanting the physiological processes associated with the symptoms of musculoskeletal dysfunction, herbs and botanicals seem to work by creating an environment where the body can bring about its own health. Furthermore, while a single drug is generally limited in scope and purpose, a single herb or botanical, with their additional ingredients, can stimulate and enhance numerous physiological processes that can have surprising therapeutic value. Although herbs and botanicals produce their effects more slowly than manufactured medicines—because herbs, according to the author, herbal proponent, and medical doctor Andrew Weil, use an indirect route to the bloodstream and organs—their primary outcome is more than a gradual abatement of symptoms. Rather, they seem to help in restoring normal function.

SIDE EFFECTS While there are some clear advantages to using herbs and botanicals in place of manufactured medications, let us not forget that they are all still drugs that can be dangerously toxic if taken incorrectly. Because we still know very little about the exact mechanism of most herbs and botanicals, many of their side effects are simply unknown. Although there have been a plethora of new studies that have considerably advanced the entire field, we have but scratched the surface, especially in an empirical collection of reliable data.

WHEN TO SAY YES With the unanswered questions about use, interaction, and risk, making a specific prescription is hard to calculate and recommend. However, I do advocate the exploration of herbs and botanicals for use in relieving or treating chronic pain in conjunction with therapeutic movements. With that said, I strongly advise that you *not* do so on your own. You should contact an alternative medical physician before proceeding with any protocol or regimen.

Diet and Nutritional Supplements

MOST COMMONLY TAKEN There are simply too many foods and nutritional supplements that directly affect the musculoskeletal system to name here. However, a selective list of those most beneficial to relieving and treating chronic pain are included in this section.

MEDICINAL KNOW-NO'S I'm sure you're well aware that having a well-balanced diet is good for you. What you may not know is that certain foods can alleviate and prevent the pain associated with musculoskeletal dysfunction while others can aggravate it. Furthermore, a nutritious diet can bolster your body's immunological processes and increase the restorative powers of your muscles and joints while others can reduce them. Nutrient-rich foods (see the following) trigger metabolic reactions that can relieve inflammation, relax muscle spasms, build stronger bones, and stimulate cartilage regeneration. While diet is not a replacement for therapeutic movements, it is a vital complement for keeping your body in optimal biomechanical condition.

Following is a prescription plan (organized to parallel our examination of medicines) for eating your way to a pain-free life.

Anti-inflammatory: Just in case you haven't already heard, saturated fats raise your bad cholesterol levels. Did you know that they can also raise the amount of bad inflammatory hormones? Foods that contain saturated fats, such as butter, cheese, cream, meat, and tropical oils, increase the production of proinflammatory

Did You Know That . . .

■ **The three leading causes of death in the United States are associated with a poor diet?**[23]

■ **Only 9 percent of all American adults consume enough healthy foods to reach the minimum recommended daily intake of nutrients?**[24]

■ **88 percent of adult Americans take nutritional supplements, of whom less than half do so regularly?**[25]

prostaglandins. Foods that contain unsaturated fats, such as flaxseed, pumpkin seeds, salmon, sardines, tuna, and walnuts (all high in omega-3 fatty acids), increase the production of anti-inflammatory prostaglandins. Thus eating unsaturated fats can help to affect the predomination of anti-inflammatory hormones over the proinflammatory ones. There is substantial evidence to suggest that altering your diet to include these good fats and exclude the bad ones is a natural and noninvasive way to reduce inflammation and relieve its accompanying pain.

Muscle relaxants: Such foods as artichokes, broccoli, nuts, spinach, soybeans, and sweet potatoes relax muscles because they contain a high content of magnesium, a mineral that plays a part in the activation of normal muscle and nerve function. Magnesium has been shown to relieve and help prevent muscular pain caused by spasms, cramps, and headaches. There are also some exciting new studies that indicate the essential role magnesium plays in combating fibromyalgia and nerve-related disorders.

Analgesics: An effective way to stimulate the production of your body's painkilling agents is to trick them into thinking you're hurt. How do you do this without actually hurting yourself? For starters you can bite into a jalapeño pepper! That's right. The brain perceives a hot, spicy food as if it were a real injury. It responds to the fiery sensation with a burst of endorphin release. As nerve receptors on the tongue adapt and the threat diminishes, the floodgates are closed. But, by the time that happens, you will already have the naturally occurring pain relief you wanted.

Bone production: Although you lose some bone mass as you age, a diet rich in calcium and vitamin D, coupled with therapeutic movements, can counteract much of the loss. Foods that contain ample amounts of calcium, which increases bone depository and production, are broccoli, leafy green vegetables, tofu, and yogurt. Foods that contain ample amounts of vitamin D, which helps the absorption of calcium into the bone, are eggs, fish, and liver. Eating these foods can make a world of difference to your skeletal structure.

Cartilage regeneration: Some people may find it ill-mannered to chomp down on chicken bones, but there is a surprising benefit to this dietary delight. Chicken bone cartilage (as well as other animal connective tissue) contains glucosamine, a naturally occurring substance that improves joint function and repair. While there is no substitute for nourishing the cartilage in your joints with their own synovial fluid, these foods can reinforce and stimulate new cartilage production. Glucosamine tablets, made from the shells of lobster, crabs, and shrimp, are a viable alternative if you find the aforementioned practice too impolite. Much has been made recently of the curative value of glucosamine supplements. Once again, I say that you will not find a cure to musculoskeletal dysfunction in a pill. However, the addition of glucosamine to your diet or in supplement can enhance the health of well-cared-for joints.

It is amazing how much improvement can be made to your musculoskeletal system by including nutritious foods, such as fruits and vegetables, in your diet. And yet studies show that most Americans do not eat the recommended allowance of five to six servings daily. The symptoms of the resulting vitamin and mineral deficiency, which have been largely ignored or misdiagnosed by many doctors, range from mild to severe. In fact, chronic nutrient deficiency has been implicated in a whole host of pain-related ailments, including muscle weakness, bone loss, and neural misfiring. So, once again, we turn to pills to compensate for the deficit we've created instead of to the foods that can bring us so much healing and health.

Food or nutritional supplements are condensed versions of the nutrients found in foods. Go into any supermarket and you will find the shelves stacked with every conceivable vitamin and mineral. While it is safe to say that walking over a few more aisles to the produce section will yield a better source of nutrients, there are legitimate reasons for taking supplements. Some people unwittingly cook the nutrients out of their foods or eat food grown in depleted soil, while others simply lack the knowledge or time to plan suitable meals. On top of this, even those with an adequate mainstay of fruits and vegetables can suffer depletion from stress, genetics, disease, and certain medications. In these instances, supplements can be a valuable way to replenish diminished nutrient levels. However, it is important to understand that supplements are not a cure-all for poor eating habits. That's why they're called supplements, not replacements.

SIDE EFFECTS It may seem silly to include a side-effects section on food, but there are some surprising studies that have shown a direct link between some foods and arthritic pain. For instance, arthritis sufferers report an increase in symptoms from refined or processed grains, flour, and sugar. Saturated fats and fried foods also exacerbate musculoskeletal pain. The good news is that if you stay away from these foods and replace them with healthy alternatives, such as whole grains, natural sweeteners, unsaturated fats, and fruits and vegetables, you may be able to reduce your symptoms.

Supplements should not be treated lightly or taken randomly. Some, if taken in large doses or for prolonged periods, can be toxic to your system. Others can interact in unexpected ways with each other and with prescription medications. They can affect people with preexisting conditions and are not recommended for pregnant or breast-feeding women unless advised otherwise. You should consult your doctor before undertaking a prescribed regimen and always take the recommended dosage.

WHEN TO SAY YES Either through diet, supplements, or both, be sure to get your daily allowance of nutrients. While my inclination is to have you obtain your nutrition naturally, supplements can effectively fill some of the gaps in your diet.

In the final analysis, if you want to have a strong, healthy musculoskeletal system, free of aches and pains, you should balance your diet and get moving properly.

Musculoskeletal dysfunction promotes an assortment of symptoms, including inflammation, muscle spasms, and pain. As I have said, drugs, and herbs and botanicals to a certain extent, are only a temporary solution. To produce more permanent change and lasting relief, you must maintain the optimal physiological environment for your muscles and joints.

Happy Endings: Gayle's Story

Gayle L., age 50, had a long history of chronic pain and dysfunction when I began treating her in 1998. Her numerous problems included a reversal of her cervical spinal curve, multiple segmental instabilities of her back, unstable posterior migration of her jaw, sacroiliac joint macrotrauma, hamstring muscle microtrauma with nerve involvement, and significant other sprains, strains, and injuries. She had also been taking a plethora of different pain medications for nearly two decades. Of all my patients, she was one of the worst cases I had ever seen.

If ever there was a hopeless case, I was it. At least that's what every health care professional I saw over a 25-year period told me. And who could disagree with them? For almost half my life, because of a series of injuries, concurrent stresses, and daily events, I lived in a body with multiple musculoskeletal problems and chronic pains. It was like a living nightmare: Every inch of my body hurt, literally from head to toe. I sought out every type of medical doctor and alternative practitioner available. Their prognosis: hopeless. I had every imaginable diagnostic test performed and even had biofeedback machines attached to my body. Their prognosis: hopeless. My condition was so bad that most of the practitioners I went to simply washed their hands of me. Having run through all of my options, being unable to function, and wanting desperately to have just a little reprieve from the constant and torturous pain, I began taking pain medications. I took over-the-counter anti-inflammatories, prescription anti-inflammatories, muscle relaxants, antidepressants, and even a few opiates. I tried every conceivable herb and botanical, including cayenne pepper, glucosamine sulfate, and feverfew. I even sprinkled turmeric on everything I ate, hoping it would help. The upshot of all those drugs? While I had some temporary moments of relief, I was still hopeless. And that's how my life remained until I went to see Dr. Weisberg.

Early on in my incredible recovery, Dr. Weisberg suggested that I wean myself from all the drugs I was taking. His reasoning was sensible and scientific: Drugs mask pain, making it both harder to obtain a realistic picture of my progress and easier for me to function under false pretenses, thus leaving me more vulnerable to re-injury. He also told me that many short-term-acting drugs actually make the healing process take longer because they inhibit the physiological processes responsible for wellness. As a nurse, I knew he was right. But I was afraid to stop.

Pain medications are bittersweet for someone in the condition I was in. While I knew deep down that they weren't doing anything to help cure my problems, they were often the only way to get relief from my misery. There were times that I honestly thought I couldn't live without them. Although I was never physically addicted to the medications (I had seen too many pain patients go down that harrowing road), I think I was psychologically dependent on them, like a crutch. But once I started to feel real, consistent relief from Dr. Weisberg's treatments, I knew that I didn't need or want them in my body anymore.

Dr. Weisberg's methods gave me my life back. He built me up slowly but surely, asking me to take an active role in my recovery. This meant doing his targeted therapeutic movements in conjunction with his daily program (customized, at first, for my condition). It also meant staying away from medications that would impede the integrity of the finely tuned healing systems that make it possible for my body to make itself well. Dr. Weisberg taught me that if I gave my body what it needs and refrained from giving it what it doesn't, then I can get better. As I started to become pain free while being drug free, I began to realize that my body was not my enemy, that it wanted to be restored to normalcy as much as, if not more than, I did.

The doctors said that it would take nothing short of a miracle for me to be well again. Dr. Weisberg said that it would just take time and work. While he was right, I still like to think of the Weisberg Way as a miracle. Five years ago I would have been satisfied to get to a point where I wasn't afraid to move. I've gotten so much more. My problems and pains are all but gone, and my activities have returned to normal and grow each day. Dr. Weisberg made the impossible possible by turning a hopeless case into a hopeful one.

5: The Earth Is Not the Center of the Universe, But the Navel Is the Center of Gravity: Musculoskeletal Myths Debunked

COPERNICUS'S PROCLAMATION that the earth was not the center of the universe challenged the accuracy of one of the most deeply ingrained and widely held beliefs of the time. Humanity is often comfortable with its myths and resistant to change its views, even in the face of overwhelming evidence to the contrary. Like the people of the 16th century who clung desperately to the false belief of the earth's central placement in the solar system, many people today cling to outdated and incorrect notions about their own bodies. And as some were shocked when Copernicus put the sun squarely where it belonged, so, too, some may be shocked to find that many of the tenets of musculoskeletal health whose truth they took for granted actually hamper their general well-being.

I wrote this chapter to debunk the myths that contribute to the advent and perpetuation of musculoskeletal pain. I am going to challenge the conventional wisdom because, as it pertains to musculoskeletal health, it is often wrong. The previous chapters provided you with all the background information you'll need to understand why these myths are false. Now we'll explore how these myths make you vulnerable to misdiagnosis and mistreatment.

From the many musculoskeletal myths to choose from, I selected the most damaging and destructive. Some of the myth busters tackle ideas and behaviors that have been with us for a long time; others address myths that are only a few years old. All of them share a common denominator: They remove the roadblocks to optimal musculoskeletal health.

Myth: **Aging is a musculoskeletal disease.**
Myth Buster: **It is possible to age gracefully.**

One of the most common myths is the idea that the human body was not de-signed to survive intact into old age. According to this myth, the aging process in and of itself brings about arthritis, limited mobility, and pain. This is a very dan-gerous premise because it leads to the erroneous conclusion that these are in-evitable conditions and thus impossible to prevent. While it is true that the musculoskeletal system loses mass and density as it ages, this alone is not enough to account for the vast number of elderly people who suffer from severe muscu-loskeletal decay and deterioration. Nor can it justify the rising number of middle-aged and young people suffering from these "age-related" health problems. In addition, it completely ignores those cultures whose people exhibit extremely high musculoskeletal health into their 80s, 90s, and beyond. But if the aging process isn't responsible for such gross musculoskeletal problems, what is?

Musculoskeletal ailments that are associated with old age are actually the re-sult of years of cumulative dysfunction and neglect. Because our lifestyle doesn't promote a healthy biomechanical existence, we incur subtle injuries from daily wear and tear. Over time, these painless microtraumas lead to tissue damage, which in turn leads to the painful destruction of cartilage, bones, and muscles. While some of us may make it through a good portion of our lives pain free, the conditions leading up to the sudden onset of pain and limited mobility are present long before they express themselves symptomatically.

Further compounding the physiological problem of accumulated muscu-loskeletal dysfunction is the psychological phenomena of aging. While many peo-ple think that the passage of time robs them of their ability to do the things they were capable of doing when they were young, it is more often the case that people slow down and become less active simply because they have gotten older. It follows that the less they do, the less they are able to do. The less able they are, the more susceptible to dysfunction. The more dysfunction they incur, the more pain they feel. The most potent way to avoid the catastrophic effects of musculoskeletal dysfunction in our later years is to care for our muscles and joints early in life. For those of you who have already entered the second half of life, here's some good news: It's never too late to start.

The musculoskeletal system is remarkably reparative and needs very little in the way of maintenance. Furthermore, the natural tendency to lose bone and muscle mass as we age can be counteracted through an increase in demand, activity, and proper nutrient intake. My program helps to neutralize many of the effects of aging and is able to bring about optimal musculoskeletal health in people of all ages because it provides for these specific needs. Arthritis, limited mobility, and pain do not have to taint your golden years. It is possible to age gracefully after all.

Myth: Pain is all in the mind.
Myth Buster: Pain is real.

Pain is one of the most misunderstood phenomena of the human experience. This is mostly because it is a subjective, intangible, and highly complex feeling. All of the traditional Western modes of analysis, including observation, dissection, and X-rays, offer very little in the way of a clear-cut diagnosis for pain. That is why chronic pain has always been such a difficult condition to treat. But over the course of the last two decades, we have seen enormous advances in the understanding of pain. Where once doctors use to disregard chronic pain, they now see it as a syndrome that demands attention and care.

One of the great scientific leaps to come out of this time is recognizing the connection between pain and the mind. The validation of this relationship opened up alternative avenues of treatment for musculoskeletal pain never before considered. Some health professionals learned how to make symptoms more tolerable by raising the pain threshold in the patient's mind. Others reduced the pain itself by working to reduce the mental states that irritate the musculature and, by proximity, the joints. Because all pain is a perception of the mind, making the mind a component of treatment has produced very beneficial results. However, there are a small but growing number of doctors who have taken this idea too far. They maintain that musculoskeletal pain is nothing more than a psychosomatic manifestation. In other words, they totally embrace the psychological element and ignore the mechanical aspects of musculoskeletal pain.

Musculoskeletal pain is a symptom of biomechanical dysfunction. While the mind can *contribute* to dysfunction—for example, stress, anxiety, and tension can cause a tightness of the musculature, which in turn imposes an additional load on the joints—it does not cause dysfunction in the first place. Although some negative mental states can exacerbate a compromised musculoskeletal system, there must be an underlying vulnerability present to begin with for them to produce pain. The truth is that a well-tuned musculoskeletal system is resilient enough to withstand most negative emotions.

The real danger in thinking that pain is all in the mind is in its corollary treatment. For example, drugs, such as tranquilizers and antidepressants, are used to quiet the mind in order to stop the ill effects on the body. But because the biomechanical aspects of the pain are virtually ignored with this approach (and others like it, such as hypnotherapy), the treatment is a temporary and symptomatic solution, not long term and therapeutic in nature. Thus the biomechanical dysfunction is perpetuated and festers as it permanently erodes the structure.

With that said, I believe very strongly in the mind/body connection. The mental and physical bodies work in tandem with each other to either impede or assist in creating a healthy human being. But without a basic level of proper musculoskeletal function, the mind will become enslaved to physical discomfort and pain. No matter how hard you try to calm and ease the mind, biomechanical dysfunction will always take precedence. It is only by embracing the physical that one can transcend it.

Myth: Genetics determine musculoskeletal health.
Myth Buster: Genetics play only a partial role in musculoskeletal health.

There is no doubt in my mind that the field of genetics is revolutionizing and re-defining our understanding of, and approach to, health-related issues. While it has been known for more than a century that superficial characteristics, such as eye and hair color, are determined by our genes, scientists are just starting to discover that many psychological traits, such as shyness, and physiological traits, such as immunization from or susceptibility to many diseases, are also determined by our genes.

One hot topic of debate in the scientific community—and our most current myth that needs debunking—is that osteoarthritis (OA) and other musculoskeletal ailments are genetic in nature. The theory postulates that some people possess a genetic inevitability or predisposition for biomechanical problems, irrespective of lifestyle, fitness level, diet, and proper musculoskeletal care. While biochemistry and the genetically determined size, shape, and strength of your bones, muscles, and cartilage most probably *influence* the physiological and functional aspects of your musculoskeletal system, they do not *determine* its ultimate health. Why? Let me illustrate with an example.

Let's say you have two cars, one that cost more than $80,000 and one that cost less than $20,000. If you drive each for 100,000 miles, oiling, tuning, and caring for only the less expensive model, which do you think will outperform the other? While the mechanical parts of the more expensive car may start out at a higher quality, they will end up performing to capacity only if the car as a whole is well maintained. All upkeep being equal, the less expensive car can last almost as long as the more expensive car if given the proper care.

The same applies to the biomechanical aspects of two individuals, one with a genetically stronger and one with a genetically weaker musculoskeletal system. If they lead similar lifestyles in terms of bodily usage but only the genetically weaker one maintains optimal biomechanical function, which do you think will end up with arthritis and pain? While the biomechanical parts of the genetically stronger individual may be less susceptible to dysfunction and daily wear and tear, this person's musculoskeletal system will eventually fail and perform to capacity only if it is well maintained. Likewise, the person with a genetically weaker system will have fewer musculoskeletal problems as long as she or he is vigilant with its care. While genetic predetermination most likely establishes the degree to which you are at risk for OA and other musculoskeletal ailments, you can alter this proclivity in either direction, making it weaker or stronger by neglect or upkeep, respectively. Therefore, your choices, more than your genetics, will determine the outcome of your musculoskeletal health.

Myth: X-rays and MRIs tell the whole story.
Myth Buster: X-rays and MRIs do *not* tell the whole story.

I once posed a simple question to an orthopedic surgeon from North Shore University Hospital in New York State. His answer surprised him as much as I thought it would. I asked, "If an X-ray or MRI were taken the day before and the day after a patient developed pain symptoms, what would you find?" He scratched his head and had to admit that the two pictures would be identical.

Why is this answer so startling? Let's assume that the radiological examination of said patient showed arthritic changes or degeneration of the bone. According to the doctor reading the X-ray, the presence of degeneration would be attributed as the sole cause of the patient's pain, barring disease or trauma. Diagnosis and treatment would follow from this radiological finding. But if it is true that the abnormality would have shown up on an X-ray the day *before* any pain symptoms arose, does the X-ray really shed light on what caused the pain? Furthermore, should we base treatment, such as surgery, medication, or injections, on radiological examinations that may not tell the whole story?

To illustrate this point further, consider that researchers at the University of California Medical School in San Francisco X-rayed 200 people with severe and recurrent lower-back pain and 200 people who had never experienced even a single bout of lower-back pain. They found that arthritic changes were present with almost the same incidence in all 400. From these results, researchers concluded that visible changes in the bone could *not* be said to independently cause back pain. What then makes arthritic changes go from painless to painful? Every human being will incur abnormalities to their skeletal structure in varying degrees throughout his or her life. If you were to randomly X-ray the joints of people over the age of 40, you would find arthritic changes in almost all of them. In spite of this, some people will go through most of their lives pain free. That is because the human structure can accommodate itself to a certain amount of abnormality. However, when the source of the abnormality, which can be overstress, overweight, and overuse or underuse, continues to irritate the musculoskeletal system, even the strongest structures will succumb to inflammation, limited mobility, and pain. Therefore, it is not the degeneration of bone alone that causes symptoms to arise; rather, it is the overwhelming accumulation of microtraumas that elicits a symptomatic response from a compromised musculoskeletal system unable to accommodate itself to dysfunction any longer. While X-rays and MRIs can be useful in helping determine how fragile and vulnerable a patient's musculoskeletal system is, a physical examination—which should follow any radiological exam—will tell you to what extent the musculoskeletal system is reacting to the abnormal findings.

I have found that more often than not pain is caused by conditions that do *not* show up on X-rays and MRIs—irritation to soft tissue, including muscles, tendons, and ligaments—rather than by conditions that *do* show up on X-rays and MRIs—degeneration of hard tissue, including bones and cartilage. In the final analysis, a complete picture of diagnosis and treatment should be based on things that cannot be seen radiologically, that is by assessing biomechanical function and determining the ability to appropriately move muscles and joints.

Myth: Repetitive movements cause pain.
Myth Buster: Repetitive movements do *not* have to cause pain.

You sit down at your computer and type an e-mail. You did the same thing yesterday, and you're going to do the same thing tomorrow. And the next day. And the day after that. At the end of a month or so, you notice that your wrist is sore. In spite of this, you continue to type your e-mails. Before you know it, the gnawing ache in your wrist turns into full-blown pain. The pain limits your ability to use your wrist, and eventually its function becomes completely impaired. At that point you go to your doctor. She or he explains that the repetition of typing day after day injured the muscles or joints or both in your wrist. Seems like a logical enough diagnosis of cause and effect. But is it accurate, or is repetitive stress syndrome (RSS) a myth?

RSS is a diagnosis that entered the medical literature within the past twenty years or so. It is a general term that, as its name suggests, states that repetition—and repetition alone—irritates such tissues as muscles, joints, cartilage, tendons, and ligaments by stressing the tissues beyond their capacity to function. The theory behind the syndrome implies that the musculoskeletal system is analogous to a mechanical device in that constant overuse will erode its parts and inevitably cause it to fail. While there is some truth to this theory, it is more misleading than accurate for three important reasons.

First, both mechanical devices and the musculoskeletal system alike benefit from maintenance. If you service your car with regular tune-ups and take care of your muscles and joints, you can greatly extend their durability and life span so that use won't degrade their performance. Second, unlike mechanical devices, the musculoskeletal system is reparative. While a car will eventually become run-down, the human body doesn't have to. Your muscles and joints have built-in mechanisms that repair, restore, and regenerate tissue from the damage incurred in daily use, provided that the biological needs of your musculoskeletal system are met daily. Third, a healthy, well-tuned musculoskeletal system is strong enough to withstand repetitive, strenuous tasks and is designed to do so for close to 120 years. On the other hand, an unhealthy, dysfunctional musculoskeletal system is vulnerable to even the most mundane tasks and will succumb to degeneration rather quickly in life. One must therefore draw two conclusions: There has to be an underlying problem with your muscles and joints for repetitive movements to produce pain, inflammation, and limited mobility and that repetitive movement itself is *not* to blame for the pain.

RSS and disorders that fall under its umbrella, such as carpel tunnel syndrome, are increasingly common diagnoses. The danger in this is that the diagnosis itself sends a message that to *use* your body is to inevitably *lose* your body. In fact, the opposite is true. The deficiency of movement, not its repetition, is what causes most chronic musculoskeletal pain. Unfortunately, I have met many misguided people who, aware and afraid of RSS, have unnecessarily cut back on much of their extracurricular activity. Even more troubling is the treatment prescribed for RSS. Because repetitive movement is seen as its sole cause, eliminating movement is seen as its only viable solution. I have encountered many people who, at their doctors urging, have quit their jobs or gone on disability after receiving this diagnosis. Does that do any lasting good?

The answer is categorically no. Not using an area of your body does not eliminate the dysfunction that made it vulnerable to repetition in the first place. While inactivity will certainly lessen symptoms initially, it actually *prolongs* the deterioration of your muscles and joints, because dysfunction is progressive. Furthermore, it is unrealistic to try to stop using a body part. Eventually you *will* use it again; when you do, symptoms will return. The only proper treatment for RSS—the only way to prevent repetitive movement from causing harm—is by diligently and consistently conditioning your overworked muscles and joints to maintain the optimal health of your musculoskeletal system.

Myth: All exercise is good for you.
Myth Buster: Some exercise can be bad for you.

There is a notion that all exercise is good for you and that the more you exercise, the healthier you'll be. From a musculoskeletal point of view, these are true statements, provided that your system is well tuned, well adapted, and well equipped to handle the exercise you engage in. The problem is that most people expect exercise to lead to musculoskeletal health. This is simply not true. Most exercises, aside from those that target the cardiovascular system, bring about muscular bulk and strength; they never address appropriate muscle length and the full lubrication of joints. In the absence of optimal biomechanical function, exercise actually exposes you to musculoskeletal harm. The more you exercise under these conditions, the more damage you'll do. That is why my office is filled with well-intentioned yet injured fitness buffs.

In order to exercise risk free, you must first prepare your musculoskeletal system. Engaging in my program *before* you work out will help ensure the appropriate biomechanical conditions that are needed for most exercises. However, no amount of preparation can counteract the harmful effects of some exercises. For instance, sit-ups put undue stress on the lumbar region of the spine and contribute greatly to a vast number of lower-back problems; head rolls push the joints in your neck beyond their normal range and can cause irritation and arthritic changes in the area; and touching your toes with straight knees puts enormous pressure on the hamstrings and lower back and can injure the discs there. Although these exercises and others are the norm for many general fitness programs, they can be extremely injurious to the musculoskeletal system and should therefore be avoided.

Evolution has enabled the human body to move about in all sorts of ways without sustaining injury from the stress placed upon it. For thousands of years, humankind led an active and physically demanding existence with few musculoskeletal repercussions. Although we have become a sitting culture, our bodies still need physical challenge and stimulation. The modern phenomenon of exercising came about as compensation for our sedentary lifestyle. Unfortunately, many exercises require us to move our bodies in new and unnatural ways. Because evolution has not had the time to play catch-up, we are structurally ill equipped to accommodate movements of this kind. Here's a little tip I give to my patients to distinguish exercises that promote health from those that impede it: *If an exercise has no correlation to the way you move your body in the real world, it is probably harmful.* Instead, it is healthier and safer to let your body be your guide to equipping your exercise regime with simple, natural movements.

Myth: Strong muscles mean a healthy musculoskeletal system.
Myth Buster: Strong muscles are *not* an indicator of musculoskeletal health.

Looking the picture of health is often equated with being healthy. When someone has a strong, well-pronounced musculature, it implies an underlying condition of musculoskeletal well-being. In fact, strong muscles imply only one thing, strength. And strength alone does not play as large a role in optimal musculoskeletal health as you may think.

Throughout my years as a practitioner, I have seen many robust body-builders and athletes who have poor biomechanical function. Conversely, I have met many people with small muscles who have optimal biomechanical function. What accounts for this discrepancy?

Musculoskeletal health is not dependent upon strength, per se, because the most vulnerable part of this system is the joints, not the musculature. Facilitation of healthy joints requires the maintenance of optimal muscle length and the full lubrication of their cartilage, because this permits frictionless, fluid movement. While weak, inflexible, and underused muscles can certainly impede function, strong muscles that do not meet these criteria can deal an even larger blow to the system because they inflict greater force on the joint. Far more important to musculoskeletal health is providing a balanced ratio of musculature around the joint so that the muscles can move it efficiently. In the final analysis, strength plus proper biomechanical function equals optimal musculoskeletal health.

Myth: **No pain, no gain.**
Myth Buster: **Pain, no gain.**

If you've ever been to a gym, had a trainer, or worked out with a friend, you've probably heard someone say, "No pain, no gain!" This popular slogan is meant to motivate and challenge you to transcend your physical limitations. The thinking is that if you don't feel pain while exercising, you're not gaining real benefit from those exercises. In theory, it's a good idea. Many people often underestimate their own physical capabilities and so end up settling for less. Here, however, less is more.

Pain is the body's natural alarm system. If an exercise causes you pain, it is a surefire warning sign that harm is being done to your body. When you ignore the pain and repeat those exercises day after day, month after month, you are actually reinjuring an already injured area. You cannot possibly gain any benefit when you're hurting yourself. Eventually, the pain will follow you out of the gym and into your life. A multitude of chronic musculoskeletal ailments are created and compounded by exceeding your body's natural limits.

My slogan is *"To* the pain, not *through* the pain." While it is always good to physically push yourself, push only to the point of pain, then back off. Use pain as a natural barometer to monitor yourself. Then you can exercise risk free and fully reap the benefits.

Myth: Heat packs should be used on an injury.
Myth Buster: Cold packs are more effective.

The most widely practiced myth on our list is applying heat packs instead of cold to an injured area. The instinct to apply heat or cold to an injured area is a good one. Whether you suffer from arthritis, headaches, a stiff neck, sore knees, swollen joints, or an aching back, temperature variation helps to stimulate and increase the healing process in a safe, nonintrusive way. But, although both heat and cold produce results by the same physiological process, cold is substantially more effective.

The body has a core temperature of around 98.7 degrees Fahrenheit. Because the body must maintain this core temperature to survive, challenging the surface of the body with a variation sends it into crisis mode and initiates counteractive measures. To protect itself from the perceived danger, blood from around the body is redirected to the source of the insult. As circulation increases, the area's extreme temperature variant is diluted and the core temperature is maintained. Although the physiological intention is one of restoration, an inadvertent benefit is an increase of vital nutrients to the area and a flushing-away of excess fluids from the area. The net result is a reduction in inflammation, pain, and other by-products of macrotraumatic or microtraumatic injury. The surface of the human body can tolerate a prolonged increase in temperature of only 20 to 25 degrees before burning, it can tolerate a 60-degree drop in temperature before getting frostbite. The greater the variation in temperature, the greater the healing.

The only time heat is more appropriate than cold is for someone who is on either end of the age spectrum (an infant or senior citizen), medically compromised (someone with a weak heart), or suffering from poor circulation or circulatory disease. In all other instances, cold should be applied for 15 to 20 minutes, because this is how long it takes the body to reflood the area with immunizing agents.

Myth: Bed rest is good for you when you're in pain.
Myth Buster: Bed rest is a surefire way of perpetuating your pain.

When you're suffering from irritating aches or debilitating pains, you first instinct is to want to lie in bed. And who can blame you? The minute your body hits the comfortable, cozy mattress, you feel your symptoms subside. Of course, while you're lying there almost completely immobile, you're likely not to feel much of anything at all. But the minute you get out of bed, your symptoms and your condition are likely to be more severe than they were before. Whatever temporary relief you may enjoy is overshadowed by the fact that protracted bed rest compounds musculoskeletal pain.

There was a time not long ago when doctors prescribed bed rest as a recuperation from, or treatment for, many acute and chronic ailments, including, but not limited to, musculoskeletal pain. While the medical community has completely revised its standing on this practice, many laypersons still self-prescribe bed rest for considerable time, only to find their symptoms mysteriously getting worse instead of better. Let's solve this mystery now by reviewing some basic facts about how the human body works.

Your body needs movement and the demand it places on its various systems to survive. Inactivity—in this case, protracted bed rest—reduces physiological demand to dangerous levels. This can have grave consequences. For instance, the lack of demand causes bones to lose calcium, which makes them brittle, weak, and more vulnerable to reinjury. The lack of demand also causes a reduction of nutrients to the muscles, which makes them lose mass, atrophy, and place additional load on the joints. Joints become stiff or stiffer and therefore do not get their full lubrication of synovial fluid. This in turn causes the cartilage to deteriorate and arthritic changes to commence and progress. Your cardiovascular system slows down. As circulation diminishes, so too does the healing process. Internal organs can fail, and blood clots can form. Protracted bed rest is so bad for you that even people who have undergone the most invasive surgery are made to get up out of bed as soon as they are able to.

While a little bed rest when you are in musculoskeletal pain—15 to 30 minutes at most during the day—won't hurt, it is important that you keep moving. Use pain as your guide to what you can and cannot do. You want the activities you engage in to bring you right up to the brink of pain without pushing past it. Mobility, coupled with therapeutic movements designed to eradicate the underlying condition, will bring about a noticeable improvement until one day you'll find that you are completely pain free. Then the only time you'll feel the need to get into bed is for a good night's sleep.

Myth: **It is best to sleep without pillows.**
Myth Buster: **Pillows are necessary for musculoskeletal health.**

In an effort to isolate the causes of chronic musculoskeletal pain, fingers have been pointed in many directions, mostly the wrong ones. Pillows got the brunt of this for a while, and even though they are no longer the focus of blame, they were left with a bum rap. Do they deserve this? Do pillows help or hurt musculoskeletal health?

Six to ten hours a day are spent in the recuperative state of rest. To receive the benefits of sleep without incurring musculoskeletal problems, you should sleep in a position that does not place demands upon the system. This means that your joints should not be bent, curved, or extended much beyond their midrange of motion so that your muscles are in a relaxed state. How do you achieve this? With a little help from your feathery friends.

Pillows do more than just provide comfort and security. By filling in the gap between the surface of the bed and your head, they create natural postural alignment. This neutral position eliminates the need for muscular contraction, which in turn alleviates any undue prolonged imposition on the joints. For instance, if you were to sleep on your side—the preferred way to sleep, from a musculoskeletal

The Perfect Pillow Test

When searching for the perfect pillow to suit your musculoskeletal needs, try this pillow test: Stand up and place your back against a wall. With your heels touching the wall, maintain a relaxed and comfortable posture. You will find that there is a gap between the wall and your head and neck. Place the pillow you are considering in that gap. If the pillow pushes your head too far forward, it is too thick. If the pillow allows your head to fall back toward the wall, it is too thin. The right pillow for you is the one that neither props your head up nor lets it tilt down. By the way, it doesn't matter if a pillow is hard or soft or made of down or foam. The most important criterion is that the pillow maintain your head in a neutral position in relation to your spine.

standpoint—or on your back without a pillow, your head would tilt sideways or and downward, or backward, respectively. Because tilting is not a natural position, it forces continual muscular contractions. After eight hours of sustained shortening of your muscles, they'll be stiff when you awake. This in turn threatens the health of your joints. In fact, it is appropriate to sleep without a pillow only if you sleep on your stomach—the worst way to sleep—because a pillow forces your head to tilt unnaturally upward. In the final analysis, pillows make it possible for your night's sleep to be therapeutically restful.

Myth: An uncomfortable chair is bad for your back.
Myth Buster: A comfortable chair is worse.

Common sense tells us to associate discomfort with something that isn't good for us. Generally, that is correct and appropriate thinking. However, when it comes to seating accommodations, the opposite is true.

A comfortable chair is potentially more harmful and destructive to your back than an uncomfortable one for a few important reasons. First and foremost, comfort promotes prolonged sitting. Sitting for 45 minutes or longer puts a damaging amount of pressure onto your lower back, hips, and knees. In fact, long bouts of sitting are responsible for the majority of chronic musculoskeletal pain in the world today.

But it's not just the duration of time seated that is destructive to the musculoskeletal system; it is also the lack of movement while seated that compounds the problem. The more static you are when you sit, the more your muscles hold on to the short, tight positions they assume to accommodate the posture of sitting. Once you get up and move around, the muscles impose an excessive load on the joints. Studies have shown that the more comfortable a chair, the less one moves while in it. Conversely, the less comfortable a chair, the more likely one is to fidget. Now I know that most of us were taught very early in life that fidgeting is bad manners. But I'm telling you that fidgeting is actually good for you. Why? Because it is a natural response to an unnatural position. Shifting around in your seat actually causes muscles to let go of their fixed positions. This in turn reduces the amount of pressure on the joints.

Finally, comfortable, cushiony chairs and couches do not support the skeletal structure or facilitate proper posture. Ultimately, optimal postural alignment while seated is a top priority because it puts the least amount of stress on the musculoskeletal system.

These points having been made, I must point out that it is possible to combine comfort with proper ergonomics. There are many companies that offer a wide spectrum of structurally supportive, aesthetically pleasing, and comfortable seating accommodations. While prolonged sitting in any type of chair is detrimental to your muscles and joints, these ergonomic chairs make a bad situation a little better. Still, for the best results, get out of your seat and move around every 45 minutes, and don't be afraid to fidget!

Myth: Health-related treatments need to be complicated to work.
Myth Buster: Simplicity is the best way to bring about optimal musculoskeletal health.

In my decades of practice, I have encountered a puzzling phenomenon time and time again. It seems that the more complicated, confusing, and complex a treatment is, the more confidence my patients have in its effectiveness. I think part of the reason for this is that we've all been sold on the idea that achieving health is a difficult, mysterious, and bewildering process. Simplicity seems to be counterintuitive to how most people envision solutions to their health problems. The less sophisticated a treatment seems to be, the less we trust its ability to heal. It's safe to say that many health professionals like it this way, even using this thinking to their advantage. And that's the reason why this myth needs to be debunked.

Simplicity plays a role in many health-related treatments but it is a vital necessity in bringing about optimal musculoskeletal health. Why? Because you do not want a cure to worsen your condition. Although muscles and joints are highly resilient, they are also highly susceptible to the types of injuries incurred through awkward or wrong bodily positions and movements. Complicated, difficult, and strenuous exercises that are supposed to target musculoskeletal dysfunction are hard to do and even harder to do correctly. This opens the door to the creation of new problems and the compounding of old ones. I have looked into many of the curative exercise programs available today and am amazed to find that most of them include positions that are so unfamiliar and cumbersome that they really shouldn't be done without supervision. At best, these programs provide little benefit. At worst, they're dangerous. Simple programs, on the other hand, are easy to do and do not stress the body. In developing the Weisberg Way, I took simplicity into account and incorporated it into my therapeutic movements. Subsequently, I created a safe program that all people can do—irrespective of body type and level of health and fitness—and equally benefit from.

Simplicity also promotes compliance. To receive any benefit from a program, you have to do it. Complicated programs are not only more likely to be done wrong, they're also more likely not to be done at all. By raising the level of difficulty, they also raise the level of frustration. It's hard enough maintaining the motivation to engage in health-related programs consistently. Why make it harder? While you never want to compromise proper care for convenience, it turns out that tending to the needs of your muscles and joints need not be a time-consuming endeavor. As you approach Part II of this book, which contains the Weisberg Way, you will find that three minutes a day is exactly the amount of time it takes to bring about optimal musculoskeletal health. Once again, simplicity wins out.

Happy Endings: Harlan's Story

Harlan L., age 42, is a lawyer who oversees the legal affairs of a large corporation. He is also an amateur athlete who engages in numerous high-performance sports. While Harlan has spent a great deal of time and energy perfecting the mechanics of his sports, he (like most athletes I've treated) has neglected to perfect the biomechanics of his body.

Despite my wife's insistence that I hang it up, I am a kid at heart and still participate in numerous sports, including tennis, basketball, football, and softball. As you might imagine, this competitive activity has resulted in numerous injuries and strains over the years. Although it takes a little longer for my body to recuperate these days, I am determined to continue my athletic career for as long as my body allows.

I was confused about the chronic nature of some of my injuries because I had always kept myself in above-average physical condition. I believed that because I was in good condition, I would be less prone to suffer injuries or, if they did occur, that my good conditioning would allow me to recover more quickly. Dr. Weisberg told me that this was a myth and indicated that the contrary may be true: that, in the absence of a well-tuned musculoskeletal system, my intense athleticism put me at risk to suffer injuries more often and more severe than the typical couch potato. I see evidence of this almost every day as I frequently walk with a limp through my office while my overweight and inactive contemporaries meander painlessly through the same corridors.

My most prolonged injury had been tendonitis in my right elbow. I am not sure whether it developed from pitching a baseball or serving a tennis ball, but this condition began during my junior year of high school and has persisted for nearly two decades. Although the pain was not something I had to deal with 24 hours a day, it arose every time I threw a ball or swung a racket. Often it was so severe that I was forced to stop playing.

A friend strongly suggested that I see Dr. Weisberg. From the outset, Dr. Weisberg understood my frustration and my need to stay competitive. Rather than recommend that I change my lifestyle or adjust my technique, he stressed the importance of targeted therapeutic movements to be done before and after playing. These movements, which did not require fancy or expensive exercise equipment, were designed to stretch and strengthen the muscles in my upper arm, shoulder, and forearm so that the strain on my elbow joint would be relieved. When asked about drugs, he told me that I could take them but that they would only mask the pain. If I wanted long-lasting improvement, I needed to optimize the health of my musculoskeletal system every day. That's when he showed me the Modified 3-Minute Maintenance Method for Athletes.

I can finally say that my elbow is pain free. While other major injuries (many of which Dr. Weisberg has helped me through) have often kept me on the sidelines, I'm happy to say my elbow is no longer one of them. Neither is the plethora of minor injuries that used to plague my life. I must admit that there are times when I disregard his advice and go right into an activity without doing the TMs or I get lazy and don't do the daily program—and I always pay the price afterward. For me, the simplicity and effectiveness of Dr. Weisberg's methods hit a home run.

Part II

The Solution Is the Weisberg Way

6: The 3-Minute Maintenance Method

Who it's for: **Everyone (ages 15 to 65)**

Goal: **To bring about and maintain optimal musculoskeletal health**

Bonus Benefits: **Prevents nearly all general and chronic aches and pains**

WELCOME! YOU HAVE ARRIVED AT the point in the book where all the information you've read thus far will be applied and turned into action—and results. If you're free of pain and want to stay that way, or if you're in pain, or have been in pain and don't want to be again, you're in the right place. I am about to introduce you to a simple, safe, and surefire daily program that, when done consistently, prevents nearly all types of chronic musculoskeletal pain.

The 3-Minute Maintenance Method is comprised of six easy-to-do therapeutic movements (TMs) that comprehensively address all of your body's major muscle groups and joints. I will guide you step by step, giving detailed instructions for how to do each TM correctly. I will explain to you which muscles and joints are targeted and which parts of the body reap the benefits. I will also show you how each of the TMs work so that you will understand why they are effective. Finally, at the end of the chapter, I will answer some frequently asked questions. Before you begin, however, there are a few important principles to keep in mind as you embark on your journey to a pain-free life.

Anytime Is the Right Time

It's not *when* you do the 3-Minute Maintenance Method but *whether* you do it that counts. In other words, there is no "right time"; the only "wrong time" is "no time." My program is equally effective whether it's done in the morning, afternoon, or evening and even if the time varies from day to day.

Fundamental to the success of my program, however, is doing it daily. *You* have to work it for *it* to work. I know from my own experience that it can be difficult to introduce a new element into your daily routine, even if it takes only three minutes a day and will vastly improve the quality of your life. Any change is hard, even a small one. That's why I advise that, at least in the beginning, you set up a regular time and stick to it. There are studies that suggest that the most lasting self-improvements are ones that have at some point become habits.[1] How do you make something a habit? Pick a time, stay fixed to it, and don't waver. In approximately 30 days, it should be fully and naturally incorporated into your life.

With that said, there may be a time that suits you more than others. For instance, one of my patients likes to do the 3-Minute Maintenance Method as soon as she gets out of bed in the morning so that she starts her day by being good to herself. Another patient likes to do the 3-Minute Maintenance Method right before he goes to bed at night because it helps him unwind after a long, hectic day. There are different biomechanical advantages to doing my program at one time of day rather than another. For instance, performing the 3-Minute Maintenance Method early in the day prepares your muscles and joints for the activities ahead; performing it later in the day heals your muscles and joints from the activities you have already undertaken. It doesn't really matter what time you choose. In fact, you can even do it twice, if you're so inclined. The only mistake you can make is not doing it at all.

Prevention, Not Intervention

This should be your mantra. Remember, it is much easier to prevent a problem than it is to solve it after it has become one. This is true of most things in life, and it is especially true of chronic pain. Musculoskeletal dysfunction, while usually complex, confusing, and costly to treat, is easy and simple to prevent. In fact, from a biomechanical point of view, prevention is absolutely imperative. Why? *Because the only way to win the war on pain is with a preemptive strike.*

As I explained in earlier chapters, chronic pain is the result of dysfunction caused by daily wear and tear to your muscles and joints. If you don't prevent the dysfunction from accumulating but rather allow it to progress unhindered, it will only worsen. As your musculoskeletal system is increasingly subjected to erosion and deterioration, the likelihood of injury increases. A lifelong struggle with pain is often the result. The 3-Minute Maintenance Method is designed to prevent the accumulation of dysfunction by the daily restoration of your muscles and joints to optimal condition.

Prevention is just good old common sense, because it is never wise to wait for things to go wrong before you deal with them. For instance, to avoid having your car fall into a state of disrepair, most of you regularly have the oil, brake pads, shock absorbers, and tires changed. Even if you don't know or fully understand how your car works, you do know that there are certain things that need to be done to maintain its upkeep. It is remarkable to me that most of you see this clearly when it comes to your automobiles, electronic equipment, and household appliances yet fail to make the connection that the same principle holds true for your body, which is, after all, also highly mechanical in nature. Rarely do you wait until you're on the side of the road calling AAA for a tow before you take your car in for a tune-up. So why wait for your body to break down before you do something about it?

I have had countless patients put off implementing my program because they subscribe to the notion, "If it ain't broke, don't fix it." You can no longer claim ignorance of the fact that in subtle, even microscopic ways, your muscles and joints are in an almost constant state of being "broke." The absence of pain does not mean the absence of problems. While some people may make it through a portion of their lives free of symptoms, behind the scenes their body is slowly losing the full capacity to function. Inevitably, the years of neglect will trigger an episode; by the time that happens, there will be a more urgent need to eradicate the pain than to resolve the underlying condition that caused it to occur in the first place. This starts the whole vicious cycle all over again. Better to fix it *before* it's "broke." I can tell you that it takes a lot more out of you emotionally, physically, and financially to treat chronic pain than it does to prevent it. Three minutes a day—180 seconds—is all that is needed to nurture and maintain the well-being of your body.

If There's Pain, Refrain

The 3-Minute Maintenance Method is designed for people of all ages from 15 to 65 in varying degrees of health and fitness levels. (For exceptions to the rule, such as high-performance athletes, pregnant women, children, and senior citizens, see Chapter 9.) All the TMs are easy to do and do not stress the muscles and joints. Initially, however, these positions may be unfamiliar to your body. Some minor discomfort is to be expected. What's more, you should feel a gentle stretch or pulling *every* time you engage the targeted area. That's normal. In fact, if any of the TMs do not challenge you in this way, try the corresponding TM for athletes in Chapter 9.

What's not normal is if any of the TMs cause you pain. Pain is always a warning sign and should never be ignored. I've already debunked the popular myth "No pain, no gain" in Chapter 5, but I must reiterate here that when you engage in *any* activity, including my program, you can push your body up to the point of pain but should not go past it. Once you cross over into pain, you can be sure that you are harming your body. Only you can determine what that point is, but when something goes from discomfort to pain, you should refrain.

If you do not have a preexisting painful condition yet feel pain while engaged in the 3-Minute Maintenance Method, do the TMs only as you far as you can up to the point of hurting. Even if you can go into only a fraction of the goal position, use it as a starting point and progress from there. In all likelihood, your mus-

cles and joints just need a little time to adjust. They may be tight, weak, or atro-
phied from years of neglect. Though these positions are not complicated or difficult, you are using your body in new and different ways. Work up to the full goal
positions over time by slowly increasing how far you push every day—as long as
you don't push into pain. Incrementally, you will see a dramatic improvement.

However, if a partial position is still painful, you may have unwittingly uncovered a festering dysfunction, or an area that may need a little extra attention. I
recommend that you immediately go to the Encyclopedia of Pain Relief (Chapter 7),
find that body part and its corresponding TM, and add it to the 3-Minute Maintenance Method. Within a few weeks of doing double duty, the pain should subside.

If you do have existing pain, you need to proceed carefully. While it is essential for you to do as much of the 3-Minute Maintenance Method as you can, you do
not want to make the situation worse by pushing your body too far. I amend the advice I just gave you as follows: If any of the TMs cause an *increase* in your pain, you
should refrain. It is important to understand that specific problems require specific
remedies. That's why I have allocated the next chapter entirely to targeted modes of
healing and rapid relief. Any time you feel symptoms in a specific area, you should
turn to the Encyclopedia of Pain Relief and add those body-part-specific TMs to the
3-Minute Maintenance Method. I have found that the people who do double duty
receive the most beneficial results the fastest.

Remember, however, that this isn't a race or a contest. It's a lifetime commitment to maintaining the biomechanical health of your muscles and joints. You
need to work with your body and let it dictate how far you can go. If you do feel
pain, let it guide you to what is appropriate. Whether you do the TMs fully or partially, you will reap plenty of benefit. Be patient with your body. As you restore it to
health, its limitations will fade away along with the pain.

It's Never Too Late to Start

Or too early for that matter. Most people are in poor musculoskeletal health. Even if
you've never had any problems or been in pain before, recent studies show that by

the time you are in your teens, many degenerative disorders have already begun their silently destructive path.[2] That fact, coupled with lifestyle and years of neglect, means there's not a moment to waste. It doesn't matter what age, gender, or fitness level you are, nor does it matter whether or not you've ever tried anything like the 3-Minute Maintenance Method before. You *can* begin today.

Many of my patients have said to me, "What's the use? Why bother with a program when the damage is already done?" Trust me when I tell you that musculoskeletal problems go from bad to worse because they are cumulative. This means that dysfunction builds on dysfunction. Before you know it, what was once a temporary and at most irritating problem becomes a chronic and disabling one. Moreover, there is a direct correlation between poor musculoskeletal health and macrotraumatic injury. The less well tuned your musculoskeletal system, the more susceptible you are to sprains and strains, falling, and breaking bones. The good news is that the opposite is true too. The healthier your muscles and joints, the sturdier, stronger, and more vital you are. Finally, while you can't completely repair severe damage and deterioration, there is evidence to suggest that many musculoskeletal anatomical elements, such as cartilage, actually regenerate under proper care. That is why there is no better time than now to start implementing a program that arrests further degeneration and prevents new problems from arising. You *can* go through life free of pain and you *can* age gracefully. So what are you waiting for?

Keep Your Eye on the Prize

Human nature is such that we need to be motivated to implement change. A lot of research into what motivates people shows that the greater the incentive and the more clearly perceived the benefit or reward, the more likely it is that one will take action.[3] Preventive health care runs counterintuitive to this because the benefits are in what you *avoid* rather than in what you receive. Of course you are receiving the absence of a health problem, and that should be reward enough. For most people, however, circumventing something's going wrong is at best an ambiguous motivational tool, especially when things are going right. Let's face it: When you are feeling good and aren't in pain, it's hard to believe that that can change in an instant. So how do you find the motivation to engage in the 3-Minute Maintenance Method daily? By keeping your eyes on the prize: *Every day you're free of pain is a gift.*

Hundreds of millions of people globally are suffering from chronic musculoskeletal dysfunction. Look around and you will see evidence of this everywhere. Perhaps a co-worker's back is out yet again. Perhaps a good friend can no longer engage in certain recreational activities because his or her knees, elbows, shins, ankles, or shoulders hurt. Perhaps you don't need to look further than a mirror to see an assortment of aches and pains staring back at you. Need more evidence? There is a higher incidence of chronic pain in children under the age of 18 than ever before.[4] And as baby boomers approach senior citizen status, the statistics on chronic pain are expected to increase exponentially.[5] If thinking about what you don't want your life to become will motivate you, it would be wise to keep these facts in mind.

The flip side is thinking about what you *do* want your life to become. Imagine it free of aches and pains. Imagine growing old gracefully without the onset of degenerative arthritis or restricted mobility. Imagine being active without injuring yourself. Imagine no back pain, headaches, or stiffness in your muscles and joints; a life lived without constantly going to the doctor, purchasing expensive ergonomic devices and equipment, undergoing invasive surgery, or taking drugs and herbal remedies to alleviate your pain. If positive reinforcement gives you additional incentive, it would be wise to keep these images in mind.

That you have picked up this book and read this far is an indication that you want to be free of pain and are motivated enough to do something about it. All you need to do now is devote a little time—and I do mean just a little—each day to maintaining the health of your precious muscles and joints. You have all the information and tools necessary. The rest is up to you. What you decide to do with three minutes a day can change your life.

The 3-Minute Maintenance Method

All human beings are fundamentally the same. We may have different body types, eye color, skin tone, but strip away the variant superficiality and you will find that on a basic physiological level we are all very much alike. Likewise, the anatomical makeup and function of the musculoskeletal system is remarkably similar from person to person the world over. And since our muscles and joints function in the same way, it follows that they can also be dysfunctional in the same way. Implicitly, then, we all share the same needs when it comes to maintaining and improving the well-being of our muscles and joints. This common denominator, or link, is why the 3-Minute Maintenance Method is so effective for such a wide variety of people.

The Triple "S" Solution

The 3-Minute Maintenance Method reinforces optimal musculoskeletal health daily while rectifying and eliminating any abnormalities the system acquires during its every day use. How does it achieve this without having to modify the manner in which you live? By using a system I developed called the Triple "S" Solution. All the TMs employ one or more of these strategies to bolster the performance of your muscles and joints while off-setting the deficiencies they incur from your lifestyle and habits. Here's how it works:

Triple "S" Solution

Stretching

Strengthening

Stabilizing

STRETCHING One of the most important ways to combat the conditions that lead to chronic pain is to keep your muscles at their optimal muscle length, or O.M.L. As I said in Chapter 3, every move you make causes a muscle to contract and shorten. To sustain a position with the least amount of energy, the muscle temporarily fixes itself in this short version by building physiological bridges in its fibers. While most bridges detach with a change in position, remnants and the resulting shortness remain. Under these conditions, muscles hang or tug on the joints rather than support them. Compromised this way, movement itself triggers a chain reaction of dysfunction causing a variety (if not the majority) of chronic musculoskeletal pains. To counteract this, prescribed muscle length must be restored daily.

Properly designed, biomechanically targeted stretches elongate muscles to their optimal length. A special organ that lives in the muscle's tendon (the golgi tendon apparatus) responds to the stretch by sending a signal to the fibers to let go of their short, fixed positions. Residual bridges are forced to detach, and the muscle is returned to its healthy, functional state. Crucial to the success of these stretches is their duration. It takes 30 seconds of continuous stretching to trigger this process. Anything less than this is simply ineffective. Anything over a minute is counterproductive because the longer the stretch, the more likely it is that the muscle will be irritated.

To facilitate the utmost benefit to your musculoskeletal system, I have kept the duration of each of the six TMs at 30 seconds for a total of three minutes. However, there is a little wiggle room in timing each TM. Anywhere between 30 seconds and one minute will produce the desired benefits. If done daily, this method fully restores muscles to their O.M.L. while taking the joints through their full ranges of motion, thus sustaining and maintaining the optimal performance and peak condition of the entire musculoskeletal system.

STRENGTHENING Every time you engage in an activity, whether of high or low intensity, the physical stress is shared by your muscles, joints, bones, tendons, and ligaments. Optimally, the burden of this stress should fall more on the muscles because they are durable and highly reparative, whereas bones and joints are prone to deterioration and irreversible damage. When you have weak muscles, the distribution of this stress shifts to the skeletal system, making it increasingly susceptible to wear and tear. When you have strong muscles, the opposite is true. The stronger the muscle, the more it is able to relieve the skeletal structure of the excess load, thereby increasing the health and longevity of your bones. In addition, strong muscles create a more balanced musculature. Remember that every muscle in your body is paired with an equal and opposite muscle. Together, they work synchronistically to affect movement. When one muscle in a pair is weaker than the other, there is unequal pulling on the skeletal structure. This damages the joints. When complementary muscles achieve optimal strength, this ripple effect of dysfunction is eliminated.

You strengthen your muscles by repeatedly contracting them. This can be done either *isotonically* or *isometrically*. Isotonic muscle contraction is motion against resistance. For instance, in weight lifting, lifting is the motion and weights are the resistance. In isometric muscle contraction, there is no motion, only force against resistance, for instance, pushing your arm (force) against a stationary wall (resistance). The 3-Minute Maintenance Method employs both isotonic and isometric muscle contraction by using and maneuvering your body weight to achieve strength. It is important to distinguish the type of strength-building that I am trying to help you achieve from the type of strength-building that most people normally think of. In the latter, exercises, such as weight training, are usually intended to build bulk. In contrast, my TMs are designed to facilitate appropriate muscular balance and potency, thus ensuring against strain, sprain, tendinitis, and other musculoskeletal dysfunction.

STABILIZING To achieve the optimal health of your joints, you need to strike a delicate balance between two extremes: immobility and instability. On one hand, you need to safeguard your joints against too little movement. My TMs accomplish this by mobilizing the joints through their full range of motion daily. This allows for their entire cartilage surface to be lubricated with all the essential nutrients required to maintain their health. On the other hand, you also need to safeguard your joints against too much movement. Every joint has a specific allocation of movement that it permits. At the same time, the anatomical elements that surround a joint restrict its movement from going beyond its normal range. When the joint capsule, ligaments, muscles, and tendons are loose and weak, a joint permits movement beyond its proper range of motion. Thus unstable, it is highly susceptible to injury. Through stretching and strengthening, my TMs individually target each physiological component that supports the joint. By maintaining its optimal functioning capabilities, the joint is stabilized. This ensures that movement is smooth, fluid, and most important, will not incur injury.

■   ■   ■

The musculoskeletal system is a dynamic system that responds appropriately to the demands placed on it. Heightened demands and challenges raise its physiological condition and capabilities, and reduced demands and challenges lower them. The musculoskeletal system is also a synergistic system in that the health of one component is dependent on the health of another. There is an intricate interdependence at work between your muscles and joints. When your muscles are short, weak, and not well balanced, the range of motion in your joints is limited. When your muscles are appropriately long, strong, and balanced, your joints are stable and enjoy their full range of motion. Because one dysfunctional muscle or joint is enough to upset the entire system, it may seem impossible ever to achieve optimal health. I'm here to tell you that it's not only possible but that three minutes a day is sufficient to produce the results you're after, namely, a pain-free life. And now that you understand how my program works, you're ready to begin.

Therapeutic Movements (TMs)

1. Bow

PRIMARY TARGETED AREAS: Spine, shoulders, hips, knees, and ankles

SECONDARY TARGETED AREAS: Elbows, hands, fingers, and shins

INSTRUCTIONS: Kneel on the floor and sit your buttocks on your heels. Your legs should be hip-width apart. Bend over and reach forward as far as you can. Place your palms flat on the ground and spread your fingers wide, keeping your arms shoulder-width apart (see 6–1). Your arms and elbows should be straight and your head should be slightly elevated in a comfortable and neutral position. Hold for 30 seconds.

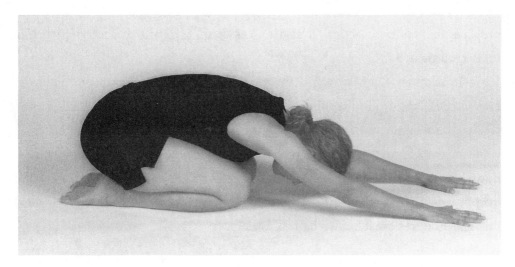

6–1. Bow

ANALYSIS: We begin with a TM that focuses on one of the most important and complex facets of human anatomy: the spine. Its optimal condition is vital to overall health because it is the foundation for the structural stability of the entire body. All activity and inactivity affects the spine because we depend on it to perform our most essential movements, including standing, hoisting the head, sitting, bending forward or backward, and rotating from side to side. Although I addressed the spine in detail in Chapter 3, I cannot stress enough that it accounts not only for so much function, but also accounts for a great deal of dysfunction. In fact, next to the common cold, back pain is the most frequent medical complaint.

The source of spinal dysfunction is our lifestyle, which neglects to take the spine through its full range of motion daily. The Bow supplements this deficiency by mobilizing the spinal joints and stretching the paraspinal muscles, the five layers of muscles that run along the spine and account for the vast majority of back pains. As you move into and hold the position, the joints become lubricated with synovial fluid and the paraspinal muscles are restored toward their O.M.L. This releases tension and tightness over the entire length of the spine, starting at its base, moving up the back, extending through the neck, and ending at the head. This TM further enhances total body performance by helping to prevent the accumulation of microtraumas in the primary targeted areas. Because the Bow finely tunes and prepares the spine for action, it also makes you less prone to acute injury and macrotrauma.

In addition, the Bow targets the muscles and joints in the upper and lower extremities. Specifically, the joints of the shoulders, hips, knees, and ankles (preventing shin splints) are in full *flexion*—the muscles bend to pull bones together, while the elbow, hands, and fingers are in full *extension*—the muscles straighten to move bones away from each other. As the muscles contract and stretch around both the primary and secondary targeted areas, they strengthen and stabilize them. Thus this TM produces great biomechanical benefit.

2. Arch

PRIMARY TARGETED AREAS: Spine, neck, wrists, hands, fingers, and abdominal muscles

SECONDARY TARGETED AREAS: Shoulders, forearm muscles, elbows, hips, shins, ankles, and feet

INSTRUCTIONS: Come to a kneeling position. Lean forward and place your palms flat on the floor underneath your shoulder, with your fingers spread wide apart. Keep your back and head straight. Slowly arch your back upward (see 6–2a), while lowering your head. Then reverse the movement. Slowly arch your back downward (see 6–2b), while raising your head. This continuous motion should take three seconds. Do this 10 times for a total of 30 seconds.

ANALYSIS: Once again we target the spine, this time focusing on activating the spinal joints through movement. The spine is made up of 24 cylindrical bones, or vertebrae. Facets, or bony projections, connect the rear sections of each vertebra to form a series of interlocking joints. As you arch upward (see 6–2a), the abdominal muscles contract and the paraspinal muscles relax in a full stretch. At the same time, each facet joint is mobilized to the extreme end of its range. As you continue

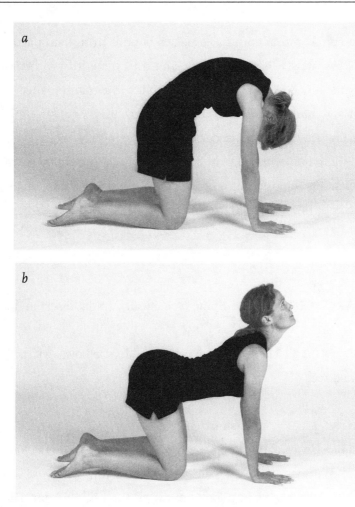

6–2a and b. Arch

the motion by arching downward (see 6–2b), the abdominal muscles relax and the paraspinal muscles contract along the spine. Once again, each facet joint is mobilized to the extreme end of its range, this time in the opposite direction. In this way, the Arch not only benefits the paraspinal muscles but also takes the spinal joints, including the neck, through their full range of motion. This ensures that the surface of the joints that connect the vertebrae are fully lubricated and nourished.

As you repeat this isotonic motion, you also strengthen your abdominal muscles. The stronger and healthier your abdominal muscles, the better able they are to carry out one of their main functions: stabilizing and supporting the lower back. As your spinal and abdominal muscles benefit from being activated, your shoulders, elbows, wrists, hands, fingers, and hips benefit from being in a supportive, fixed position. As the muscles that facilitate the maintenance of this position isometrically contract around these joints, they are strengthened and stabilized. Finally, the stretch that occurs at the ankle joints benefits the muscles of the shins and the joints of the feet, and the stretch that occurs by spreading your fingers apart benefits the muscles and joints of the wrists, hands, fingers, and the anterior muscles of the forearms.

3. Lizard

PRIMARY TARGETED AREAS: Spine (specifically, spinal discs) and lower back

SECONDARY TARGETED AREAS: Neck, shoulders, elbows, wrists, hands, fingers, ankles, and feet

INSTRUCTIONS: Lie on your stomach. Place your palms flat on the floor just wider than shoulder-width apart and spread your fingers wide. Bend your ankles so that the pads of your toes are on the floor. Slowly push your head and shoulders up until your elbows are straight, and look up toward the ceiling. Your palms should end up approximately two to four inches in front of your torso (see 6–3). Keep your lower stomach touching the floor throughout. Hold for 30 seconds.

ANALYSIS: With the Lizard, our focus shifts from the spinal joints of the vertebrae to the protective cushions, or discs, that lie between them. Disc problems are responsible for an enormous amount of chronic pain. A "slipped disc" is an all-encompassing name for a condition that occurs when the contents of the disc extend beyond their normal boundaries. Lifestyle, specifically prolonged sitting and bending over; neglect; and physical stress may cause the discs in the lower back to protrude, bulge, herniate, even to rupture. Unfortunately, minor disc dysfunction usually goes unnoticed until it's too late and the disc is permanently damaged. That

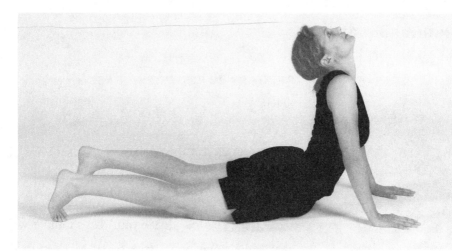

6–3. Lizard

is why this TM is so important. It not only prevents disc and lower back dysfunction, it also helps to identify and uncover hidden problems along the entire spine.

Prevention of disc dysfunction occurs as the spine is stretched in extension and the pressure pushes the discs back toward their normal position. If this causes you mild pain, you may have uncovered a minor dysfunction. In this case, you should modify the TM by bending your elbows to reduce the stretch or by bringing your bent elbows and forearms completely to the floor and fully supporting your weight on them. As you daily gradually increase the stretch, the condition will heal. Many of my patients have been spared invasive back surgery by their dedicated application of this TM. However, it is important to note that the inability to do this position without extreme pain may be indicative of a more severe disc problem. In this case, you should consult a health professional.

The Lizard also targets your ankles and feet by stretching them in the opposite way that you did in the Bow. In the latter you bent your ankles downward *(plantar flex)*; in this TM you stretch them upward *(dorsi flex)*. It stretches the front muscles of your neck, making its corresponding joints aligned. Finally, the muscles of your shoulders are strengthened and the joints of your shoulders, elbows, wrists, hands, and fingers are stabilized as the muscles around them contract isometrically.

4. Natural Squat

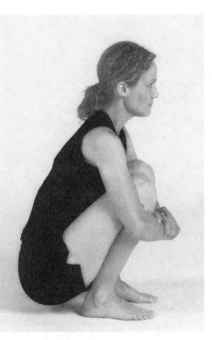

6–4. Natural Squat

PRIMARY TARGETED AREAS: Lower back and pelvis

SECONDARY TARGETED AREAS: Hips, leg muscles, knees, and ankles

INSTRUCTIONS: Place your feet shoulder-width apart and squat down (see 6–4). Make sure that your heels are flat on the floor. You may keep your arms in any position—for instance, bent around your knees as shown or straight out in front of you—but do not use any external devices for balance. Hold for 30 seconds.

ANALYSIS: In Chapter 2, I showed you how the shift from squatting to sitting in chairs is chiefly responsible for the current pandemic of chronic pain. We saw how people in cultures that still regularly engage in the simple and natural squatting position go through life gracefully, free of the vast array of limitations and pain from which most people in our society suffer. I cannot overstate how important it is to offset the lifestyle deficit of sitting in chairs. If you need a reminder, take note of these statistics: Back pain is the leading cause of disability in Americans under the age of 45,[6] and 4 out of 5 American adults from the ages of 20 to 64 will have back pain during their lives.[7] Furthermore, surgeons will perform more than 270,000 total knee replacements and 170,000 artificial hip implants this year alone.[8]

The Natural Squat can help to prevent nearly all of these. It stretches the entire lower back and reduces stress on the discs in that area. It also stretches the entire pelvic area, permitting its functional relationship with the hips and benefits the hips, knees, and ankles by putting them into full flexion. In addition, the extreme place-ment of these joints takes them through their full range of motion. Finally, as you lower yourself down into the Natural Squat, maintain it, then raise yourself up and out of it, your leg muscles (specifically, the quadriceps and gluteus maximus muscles) will be in full contraction, which adds to their overall strength.

5. Split

PRIMARY TARGETED AREAS: Hips, inner thigh muscles, groin region, and knees

SECONDARY TARGETED AREAS: Lower back, hamstring muscles, and feet

INSTRUCTIONS: In a standing position, spread your legs as far as you can while keeping your feet parallel (see 6–5a). Hold this position for 15 seconds. Next, bend at your waist and lean forward as far as you can, keeping your knees straight (see 6–5b). Your hands may touch the floor but don't have to. Hold this position for 15 seconds.

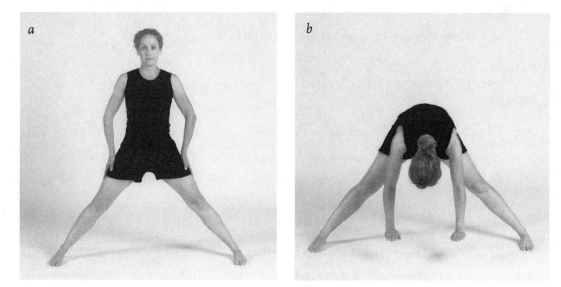

6–5a and b. Split

ANALYSIS: By design, hips are meant to open up in abduction (the moving of the legs away from the body), but our lifestyle affords them little opportunity to do so. Furthermore, the muscles of the inner thighs are meant to be challenged daily; they too suffer from underuse. Thus the knees and hips pay a hefty price, as is evident by their being the first and second most common joint-replacement surgeries each year. The Split corrects these deficiencies by stretching the muscles of the inner thigh and groin areas. As the adductor and the hamstring muscles elongate toward their O.M.L., there is a reduction of microtraumas imposed on the knees. As you maximize and maintain their health with the Split, the knee joints will be able to handle all sorts of activities, including walking, jogging, running, and playing sports, without suffering injuries to the knees.

When you bend forward at the waist, the Split mobilizes the hips. This not only increases the health of these vital joints but also stretches the musculature of your lower back. Finally, the bent position stretches the lateral muscles of the legs, which are responsible for the movement of the feet.

6. Sky Reach

PRIMARY TARGETED AREAS: Spine (specifically, proper postural alignment), shoulders, forearm muscles, elbows, wrists, hands, and fingers

SECONDARY TARGETED AREAS: Hips, knees, ankles, feet, and toes

INSTRUCTIONS: Assume a comfortable seated position on the floor with your legs crossed, and curl your toes. Interlace the fingers of your hands. Keep your spine straight and lift your arms up and over your head. With palms facing up toward the sky, reach as high as you can (see 6–6). Hold for 30 seconds.

ANALYSIS: Our final TM focuses on posture. Poor posture, or the improper alignment of the spine, is a mainstay of modern culture and adversely affects the health of the entire body (for more on posture, see Chapter 7). The Sky Reach restores optimal posture by stretching and straightening the spine. To maintain this position, the paraspinal muscles must be strong enough to hold their elongation for 30 seconds. Increasing the strength of these muscles makes it possible to carry yourself properly through the day.

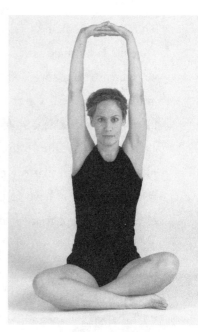

6–6. *Sky Reach*

The Sky Reach also targets the upper extremities, whose biological needs are rarely served by lifestyle. Because the upper extremities are involved in almost all activity, they are highly prone to injury. They have been addressed either directly or indirectly throughout the other five TMs; we give them extra attention here. The Sky Reach stretches the muscles of the shoulder area, including the rotator cuff muscles, thus restoring their O.M.L. while taking the shoulder joints through their full range of motion. This position also stretches the forearm muscles, which serve the elbows, wrists, hands, and fingers, while taking the wrists through their full range of motion. This TM prepares the upper extremities for virtually all daily tasks.

When you sit cross-legged in the Sky Reach, the quadriceps that cross the knees are stretched in full flexion, the dorsi flexor muscles of the ankles are stretched in plantar flexion, and the toe extensor muscles of the feet are stretched in full flexion. Finally, the internal rotator muscles of the hips are stretched in an external rotation. When these muscles are not at their O.M.L., they impose high friction on the joints, which in turn leads to arthritic changes in the hips. By doing this simple TM, you eradicate one of the main causes of the need for hip and knee replacement surgery.

■   ■   ■

That's it—you're all done. In just three minutes you have lengthened and strengthened all your major muscle groups and fully lubricated all your major joints. We started with your spine, which affects the health of your neck, upper and lower back, and shoulder area. We moved on to the hips and lower extremities, including your knees, shins, ankles, and feet. And we ended by reinforcing the health of your upper extremities, including your shoulders, elbows, wrists, hands, and fingers. Many people are surprised that my program is so simple. They have this notion that health-related programs have to be long, arduous, and painstaking (if not painful) to be effective. Perhaps that's because many of the available books and remedies are difficult and laborious. But they don't have to be, and they shouldn't be. The harder and more complex the method, the more likely it is that you will hurt—not help—yourself. All your muscles and joints need is to be taken to their full potential once a day to ensure their long-lasting optimal health.

I have been in private practice for more than 30 years and have treated tens of thousands of patients. Because I have always considered feedback to be of vital importance to my work, I began keeping track of my patients' questions regarding my program. As it turns out, there are some questions that come up often enough that I anticipate you may have them as well. I include answers to them now so that you will have a complete and clear understanding of the 3-Minute Maintenance Method.

Frequently Asked Questions

What happens if I skip a day or two?

It's safe to say that you wouldn't dream of letting a day or two go by without brushing and flossing your teeth. Aside from the obvious hygienic concerns, you are probably well aware of what can happen to your teeth if you don't regularly care for them. The same holds true for your muscles and joints. They are constantly at risk from overuse or underuse, aging, injuries, and wear and tear. Why add neglect to the list? Remember, *maintaining the optimal condition of your musculoskeletal system is a lifelong process.* There is never a time when you graduate from my program. The application of the 3-Minute Maintenance Method is a daily means of transformation and restoration to health.

With that said, skipping a day or two here and there will have little physiological effect on the structure and function of your body. However, there is a far more substantial psychological effect. Positive self-improvements are difficult to turn into habits and are easy to deviate from. We find all sorts of reasons to deprioritize our own health. Usually the excuse is lack of time. Remember, I'm not asking much of you here. Three minutes a day is not a lot of time to set aside, especially when *giving so little gets you so much.* The important consideration is that once you set a precedent for missing a day, you are more likely again to miss a day. One day turns into two, two into a week, and a week into a month. At that point you have threatened the health of your musculoskeletal system and are once again at risk for injury and pain. Better to make the 3-Minute Maintenance Method an essential and mandatory component of your daily routine. After all, what could be more important than giving yourself the gift of a pain-free life?

Should I do the TMs in order?

Yes, you should do them as prescribed. When I designed my program, I took a look at the vast majority of biomechanical dysfunctions and came up with a specific formula to counteract them. I took into account not only how muscles and joints are at risk but the way in which the different muscles and joints relate to each other in terms of repair and restoration. My program systematically and methodically works through all parts of the body in a calculated fashion. I start with the Bow because it is the foundation of body readiness from which all the other TMs build on. Think of the program as an instruction manual or recipe in which the completion of the first step is necessary for proceeding to the next. That said, you will not hurt yourself by doing them in a random order. But if you're looking to maximize the benefits, you should trust the wisdom of doing them as presented.

Do I need to do the 3-Minute Maintenance Method if I exercise regularly?

People who are very active need my program as much as—if not more than—those who are inactive. In fact, athletes and exercise buffs are more at risk and more prone to injury than couch potatoes. While it is true with regard to the body that if you don't use it, you'll lose it, it is also true that if you overuse it, you'll lose it. Let me illustrate why this is so with an analogy to an automobile.

A car that is used to haul around heavy cargo, loaded with passengers, or taken for long-distance drives is more likely to be damaged than a car that primarily sits in a garage. Although atrophy and age weaken the car that is rarely used, it requires less maintenance than the car that is subject to regular wear and tear. This is true of most mechanical devices, including your body. To exercise risk free and obtain the wonderful benefits that regular exercise provides, you must prepare your body mechanics for the rigors of use. That is where my program comes in. I designed it to facilitate overall biomechanical health.

Some of my patients have asked me why they continue to have episodes of chronic pain even though they participate in exercises that seem to do what the 3-Minute Maintenance Method does. For instance, they stretch regularly at the gym or take yoga classes a few times a week. The reason is that these disciplines were created not to restore biomechanical health but to build flexibility, endurance, and strength. Although the physical sciences have been around for close to 5,000 years, it is only in the last 50 or so that we have learned how to manipulate the body with biomechanical health in mind. I built upon the foundation of past knowledge, integrated it with current innovations, and created a simple yet revolutionary new approach. So while the body positions of other disciplines may bear a resemblance to my program, the applicability of those positions are different in some fundamental ways.

One of the most significant differences between other exercises and the 3-Minute Maintenance Method is the duration of the movements. As discussed earlier in the chapter, this is of vital importance. For instance, I have one patient who stretches his legs every day, but, because he holds this position for only 10 seconds, it has made little difference to his musculoskeletal health. I have another patient who has recurrent pain in her arms. We traced the source of her problem to yoga positions that require her to sustain a difficult pose for a minute or more. Another distinguishing characteristic of my program is its repetitive nature. It is absolutely crucial to reinforce proper mechanics of all the different muscles and joints daily. Yet most people work out by targeting one body part at a time: arms one day, legs the next, and so on. Many exercise classes do the same. Also, it is the combination of positions, the systematic and comprehensive nature, and the practically that further separates my method from other approaches.

My program is not designed to replace exercise but to complement it. There are enormous benefits that you receive from cardiovascular exercises, weight training, yoga, martial arts, and other sports that my program does not provide. What it does provide is the ability to engage in these or any other type of recreation or vocation that you choose with minimal risk of injuring yourself. The 3-Minute Maintenance Method, done in conjunction with exercise, allows for demanding activity to enhance your life, rather than diminish it by being a source of pain.

How long does it take to feel results?

You will start to reap biomechanical benefits the very first time you do the 3-Minute Maintenance Method. The positive effects are absolutely immediate. However, you should not expect to *feel* these immediate results. Just as dysfunction happens unnoticed, so too does restoration to function.

That said, you can expect to feel the manifestation of musculoskeletal health in a very short time. One of the first things you're likely to be aware of is how much more relaxed you have become. Short, tight muscles not only inhibit movement and make you prone to injury, they also create tension throughout your body. When you stretch these muscles, you release and diffuse this tension. The less tense you are, the more relaxed you feel. This effects you both physiologically and psychologically. Gradually you will begin to notice an enhancement of your well-being. As your circulation increases, an abundant supply of oxygen reaches a greater proportion of your muscles and joints. This makes you feel more vital and alert. As your flexibility and balance improve, you will feel less clumsy and more in control. And as your body becomes more finely tuned, you will feel confident in your ability to enjoy a wider spectrum of activities. I have had many patients who were under virtual house arrest because of their chronic pain. Within 3 to 6 months of beginning my program, they went from being spectators in the game of life to being participants. Most important is what you *won't* feel as a result of my program, namely, pain. The whole point of the 3-Minute Maintenance Method is to have you awaken to the idea that the aches and discomfort that you have grown accustomed to can disappear from your life. In their place, a whole new world of pain-free possibilities is waiting to be discovered.

Happy Endings: Matthew's Story

Matthew J., age 47, is a very busy lawyer. He also expends a great deal of effort keeping in shape by engaging in aerobics and weight training five times a week. In spite of his apparently excellent physical condition, he suffered from recurrent aches and pains in many areas of his body. Four years ago I treated him for one of these problems, which I diagnosed as symptomatic of dysfunctional muscles and joints.

Before I met Dr. Weisberg, my general attitude toward pain was to let it run its course. Even though some bouts would last longer than others, the symptoms would eventually dissipate. While some of my minor aches and pains ran from inconvenient to intrusive, the "time heals all wounds" method was very effective for a long time. That is until I had pain in my right shoulder.

I first noticed the pain upon arising one morning and assumed it was the beginning of a stiff neck from sleeping in an awkward position. The pain was initially nothing more than a dull ache, but it became progressively worse and more disabling with each passing day. It radiated from deep within the trapezius muscle toward the deltoid. I couldn't relax my shoulder and let my arm hang normally without going through the roof. Although it was a familiar pain (one that I had felt many times before), I had never experienced it this severely. Time did absolutely nothing to change the situation.

I tried the usual home remedies: heat, hot baths, Tylenol, and so on. Nothing

I did provided the slightest bit of relief. As the situation worsened, so did my attitude. How could pain that seemed to come out of nowhere make me so irritable and miserable? Although I knew I needed to do something more than wait it out, I didn't feel that traditional outlets provided viable solutions. My primary care doctor (whom I had seen before for pain) recommended medication and surgery, both of which were not for me. I was also a nonbeliever in physical therapy programs and exercises and had little time for prolonged treatments. I became resigned to feeling that nothing was going to help. Friends referred me to Dr. Weisberg, but I procrastinated, delayed, and made excuses until the pain was adversely affecting my sleep. With nothing left to lose, I begrudgingly sought out his advice.

On my first visit, it took a few short minutes for Dr. Weisberg to isolate the root of the problem. The ultrasound and massage therapy he performed reduced my symptoms immediately. At the end of my visit he provided me with some targeted therapeutic movements to perform multiple times over the next week. I loved these TMs because they could be done anytime and anyplace. I even did one of the movements while sitting in bumper-to-bumper traffic. Others could be performed while I sat at my desk or stood in the shower. The best part was that they worked. The treatment was nothing short of miraculous. As the days went by, the pain melted away.

By the time of my second (and last) visit, the pain was gone. At the end, Dr. Weisberg showed me the 3-Minute Maintenance Method. He explained to me that my shoulder pain and also my many other aches and pains, were the result of a less-than-optimal musculoskeletal system. Although I work out often, it seems I did little to protect my muscles and joints. Truth be told, I didn't know I had to. But I definitely felt the effects of improper maintenance. Dr. Weisberg told me that the daily program would help my body help itself to be well, whether I was active, as I was at the gym, or sedentary, as I was at the office. And he was right. Although I started out being able to do some of the TMs only half way, my ability to progress was a sign that my musculoskeletal condition was getting better. Since then, I have done this easy and effective program religiously and have remained completely pain free. I no longer have to wait for time to heal my wounds because the 3-Minute Maintainence Method prevents them from occurring in the first place.

7: Encyclopedia of Pain Relief

Who it's for: **Anyone with pain in a specific body part**

Goal: **To rapidly relieve pain in that area**

Bonus Benefits: **Prevents recurrence, reverses the underlying condition, and strengthens the area**

WHEN YOU'RE IN PAIN, the only thing that seems to matter in life is how to get out of it, fast. And with good reason. Pain is the great equalizer. It strips away all pretensions of individual uniqueness and ability and reveals our common physical limitations. The intellect cannot reason with it, the spirit cannot transcend it, and the body cannot tolerate it. Whether you are now in pain or if you're in the midst of a temporary reprieve from a chronic condition, you need not suffer anymore. The Encyclopedia of Pain Relief will provide you with the rapid relief and healing you so desperately want and need. This chapter consists of specific body-part therapeutic movements (TMs) that treat musculoskeletal dysfunction and trauma from head to toe. Included is a list of body parts and their most predominant symptoms to check against your own, detailed explanations of what brought them on, and how best to make them go away. This chapter also targets the most prevalent musculoskeletal disorders, such as carpal tunnel syndrome and sciatica; addresses many commonplace injuries, such as sprains, strains, and most of the "itises"; and rectifies poor posture. Best of all, it brings about lasting and permanent relief by eliminating the conditions that cause pain to occur and recur. However, before you begin to use the targeted modes of healing, there are a few key concepts that you need to understand so that you may proceed effectively and safely.

You Hurt Because You're Hurt

The first step on your road to recovery is recognizing that you hurt because you've hurt yourself. It may seem that this is stating the obvious, but I can assure you it's for good reason. The overwhelming proliferation, progression, and perpetuation of musculoskeletal pain is largely due to a failure to respond quickly and appropriately to its onset. Because musculoskeletal pain is rarely accompanied by obvious visual symptoms, such as bleeding or bruising, it is rarely perceived or treated as an injury. Yet that is exactly what has occurred. Specifically, symptoms such as pain, bodily noises, and stiffness are clear indications that your musculoskeletal system has been traumatized in some way. While the word "trauma" tends to conjure up images of ambulances and emergency rooms, in the world of your muscles and joints, traumas can be infinitely subtle yet nonetheless severe. Musculoskeletal traumas run the gamut from macro to microscopic:

MACROTRAUMATIC injuries are the result of sudden high-force incidents that cause damage to the soft tissue, which include muscles, ligaments, tendons, and joints. (Please note that hard-tissue macrotraumas, such as broken or fractured bones, dislocated joints, and lacerations, usually require direct medical assistance and are beyond the scope of this book.) Twisting your ankle while walking, straining the muscles in your lower back while lifting something heavy, and spraining your wrist joint when you use it to brace a fall are all examples of macrotraumas. If your pain is the consequence of a single event, you need to reduce the severity of the initial acute symptoms, such as superficial swelling and inflammation, before trying to heal the damaged tissue. Start with my 7 Steps to Immediate Relief (page 153) for a week, then proceed with the appropriate TMs in this chapter.

MICROTRAUMATIC injuries are the result of slow, continuous irritation that damages hard and soft tissue. Arthritis, cartilage and bone deterioration, limited mobility, and pain due to biomechanical dysfunction, such as short, tight muscles and underlubricated, motion-starved joints, are prime examples of microtraumatic accumulation. The vast majority of musculoskeletal pain is caused by microtraumas, injuries that are insidious because they happen imperceptibly. By the time you feel symptoms, their buildup has progressed considerably. While the 3-Minute Maintenance Method and the 3-Month Tune-Up are expressly designed to stop the silently destructive evolution of microtraumas, some things, such as lifestyle, profession, and genetics, leave you vulnerable to their onset. If your pain is recurrent, related to movement, or not the result of a single traumatic event, you need to proceed with the following TMs, as appropriate, immediately.

Macro and microtraumatic injuries are not contracted; they are acquired. This means that they come about because of something you did or didn't do, with or to your body. They can therefore (unlike many diseases) be fully healed and, more important, prevented. The musculoskeletal system has the ability to make it through an entire lifetime relatively pain free. Though as a physical and active being you are always at risk for injury, you can reduce your susceptibility by strengthening your muscles and joints. The foundation of this strength is ridding your anatomy of the destructive injuries that continue to plague it.

Relief Is a Process

In our fast-paced world we have come to expect instantaneous results, never more than when it comes to relieving pain. A $100 billion painkiller industry has sprung up around our insatiable appetite for quick fixes. Judging from the rise in chronic pain statistics, these remedies fix nothing at all. While drugs and other symptomatic treatments may give you instant gratification, it is only temporary. In fact, there is ample evidence to suggest that in the long run the false sense of security they provide prolongs and compounds musculoskeletal pain. The lesson in this is that relief should be measured not by the elimination of symptoms but by complete restoration to normalcy and health. Only a slow, gradual therapeutic process brings about lasting relief, because it unfolds as healing progresses.

Musculoskeletal pain seems to come out of nowhere, but this is a physiological illusion. In truth, it can take years, even decades, of neglect, abuse, and trauma to create the conditions that result in pain. While it doesn't take years or decades to reverse, it realistically can take weeks or months to undo the cumulative damage to your muscles and joints. You should expect relief after two to six weeks of consistent, daily single applications of the following TMs. You can expect the recovery process to be even more rapid with multiple daily applications. (Note that you should wait at least 30 minutes between applications so that the targeted muscles and joints can recuperate from and appropriately respond to the TMs.) If you're over 50 or your injury is more pronounced and has a long history, it may take a bit longer. To best guide you, I have provided in the Remedies section of each body part what short-term effects you should expect in the first week and what long-term effects after three weeks. While every person's recovery process is unique, depending on the severity of the injury, pain threshold, age, and genetics, it is important to remember that these TMs bring about relief that reflects true health. However, if you don't feel change in the allotted time, you should consult a health care professional.

To the Pain, Not Through the Pain

In the last chapter I advised that if at any point during a TM there's pain, refrain. Since the TMs in this chapter are designed to relieve symptoms, this means that you come to them with pain already present. Because of this, you must proceed carefully and cautiously. When you begin, do the TMs up to the point of pain but not past it. In other words, the moment you feel an increase in your symptoms, stop and hold that position for 30 seconds. With each successive daily attempt, push a little farther toward the goal position until your symptoms are completely gone. Continue doing the TMs for an additional two weeks after that time to ensure that the area is completely healed.

The pictures and instructions that accompany each body part TM represent the ideal positions that you will work up to over the course of your healing. Initially you may be able to do only a fraction of the total movement. That's okay. Your pain and limitations are the most accurate indicators of what your body can and cannot do. Use them wisely and be aware of your progress. Little by little and day by day, you will get closer to the goal positions as your body draws nearer to being whole and well.

Therapeutic Movements (TMs)

"Itises"

SYMPTOMS: Inflammation, swelling, pain, limited mobility

INSTRUCTIONS: For the appropriate TMs, go to the specific body parts that exhibit symptoms.

CAUSE: If you have musculoskeletal pain, you probably have one or more of the itises. That's why I start with them. Every body part and its corresponding muscles, joints, ligaments, and tendons (among other anatomical elements) is susceptible to their onset, as are all people. *Time* magazine recently stated that we are living in the Age of Arthritis, and cited it as the most prevalent itis of all. Approximately 40 million Americans suffer from this crippling condition. Another 30 million suffer from a host of others; they include bursitis, synovitis, and tendinitis.[1] Itises are the most common musculoskeletal disorders. They are also the most misunderstood, misdiagnosed, mistreated, and among the most feared. What is an itis, and what causes its appearance in so many people?

Almost all musculoskeletal pain is the result of a macrotraumatic or microtraumatic injury, and almost all macrotraumatic or microtraumatic injuries result in the occurrence of an itis that is not disease related. Itis is the Greek word for "inflammation," and the prefix used with it denotes the inflamed part. For example,

7 Steps to Immediate Relief

1. PINPOINT THE EXACT SOURCE OF YOUR PAIN

To relieve pain, you need to pinpoint and focus on its precise location. Be specific, not general.

2. STOP USING THE PAINFUL AREA

Pain may interfere with your ability to function. This is nature's way of getting you to stop using the injured area until it has had time to heal. Let pain be your guide and immediately heed its warning.

3. APPLY A COLD PACK TO THE AREA

One of the most effective ways to reduce superficial inflammation and stimulate the healing process is by putting cold on the surface of the body. (See page 113 for more.) It is important to leave the cold pack on for 15 to 20 minutes.

4. GENTLY MASSAGE THE AREA

A small amount of direct stimulation works to alleviate spasms and inflammation because it helps to relax muscles and increases the flow of circulation to the area. Be sure not to apply too much pressure. Gentle massage should bring about the desired change.

5. GENTLY STRETCH THE AREA

Stretching is a great way to immediately reduce stiff, tight, or spasmodic muscles. While you want to effect a small application of sensation, be sure not to stretch the area so much that pain results. As with step 4, being gentle is key.

6. MINIMIZE USE UNTIL HEALING OCCURS

While the first five steps will provide the relief you're looking for, remember that you are still nursing an injury back to health. Keep use of the injured area to an absolute minimum for a short time after your symptoms abate. Your body is well equipped to let you know when it is appropriate to resume normal activity.

7. PROCEED TO THE THERAPEUTIC MOVEMENTS

This is the most important step. The therapeutic movements in this chapter are designed to bring about relief by rectifying the underlying condition and syndrome of physiological neglect that brought about your pain in the first place.

tendinitis is the inflammation of a tendon. Inflammation is the immune system's natural and *healthy* response to an injury. When an injury occurs, blood vessels dilate to allow for an increased flow of nutrients and enzymes to the affected area. While the itis, or the increase in cells, proteins, and immunological fluids, causes swelling and discomfort, these resulting symptoms are the body's way of inhibiting use of the area until the healing process is complete. Normally, this process is very short: about 7 to 10 days from the initial injury. As the injury heals, the inflammation subsides; so too does the pain. Sometimes, however, the inflammatory process continues in a musculoskeletal area. In a joint capsule, it results in capsulitis. Eventually the excessive and overwhelming influx of fluids causes the area and its surrounding tissue to painfully erode and deteriorate. Why doesn't the inflammatory process turn off in these instances? What makes it go from helpful to hurtful?

Inflammation is the body's effort to resolve a crisis, and this vital process will not stop until the resolution, or healing, is complete. With a macrotrauma, the injury is so obvious and pronounced that the body's curative response is aggressive. Thus inflammation lasts for the proper and predictable time period. With a microtrauma, however, the injury is so subtle and ambiguous that the body's curative response is minimal at best. Because microtraumas are ongoing and cumulative, their daily and continual irritation triggers a daily and continual inflammatory process. Only when the source of the irritation is gone will the chronic inflammation dissipate and the process by itself return to normal.

REMEDY: Most itises are preventable. That's because most itises, especially chronic ailments such as arthritis, are caused by microtraumatic injuries. For this reason, all the following TMs target the primary cause of microtraumas: biomechanical dysfunction. Once function is restored, your itis will diminish dramatically. If you catch it early, the TMs rapidly bring relief. In the long term, they will help to circumvent lasting anatomical changes. If you have suffered from an itis for a considerable time, relief may take months. However, the TMs will stop further progression. For those of you who already have permanent damage in an area, this does not mean that you will have permanent symptoms. Your body has a remarkable ability to adapt to changes as long as its strength and health is optimally maintained. I suggest you include the TM for the body part where the itis is located in your daily routine indefinitely.

Headaches

SYMPTOMS: Mild to severe pain in the head, face, or neck region; dizziness; nausea; blurred vision

INSTRUCTIONS: Lie on the floor with your head supported by a pillow. From this starting position, lift your head and shoulders up and off the pillow. Keep your arms on the floor by your sides, and curl only your head in toward your body. Stop when your chin rests lightly on your upper chest (see 7–1). Look directly at your toes. Hold for 30 seconds. Repeat this TM daily until your symptoms are completely relieved.

CAUSE: Hundreds of millions of people around the world suffer from severe, chronic headaches. Most of those who have debilitating episodic flare-ups also endure low-grade, daily headaches. As anyone who has had one knows all too well, a

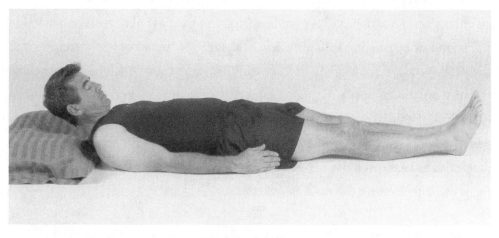

7–1. Headaches: Postural Strengthener

bad headache can be as incapacitating as the worst backache. While conventional treatments, such as medication, may temporarily ease the pain, they do nothing to bring about permanent relief.

What causes headaches? More important, what causes them to recur? Generally speaking, there are three types of headaches: migraine, cluster, and tension. Much debate and mystery surround the cause of migraine and cluster headaches. Both are thought to be either hereditary, related to gender, or neurovascular. Tension headaches are most common. As their name suggests, they are caused by the tension of musculature in the head, face, and neck regions. Although there are hundreds of known reasons why the musculature becomes tense, it boils down to one main trigger: poor posture. Poor posture, more specifically the misalignment of the head in relation to the spine, is the main factor in bringing on tension headaches—it also contributes to the onset of migraines and clusters—because it compromises the function of the upper region of the body.

The head is perched high atop the human structure in a constant battle with gravity. With optimal posture, the head easily wins the battle. With poor posture, gravity takes over and, in an effort to keep the head horizontal, forces the muscles in the back of the neck and/or at the base of the skull to continuously contract. These excessive contractions, or muscular tension, produce spasms, which painfully compress the nerves running through the neck to the head. Muscular tension can also produce pain by restricting the flow of oxygen-rich blood to the region or by causing inflammation at the site of the muscular attachment to the skull. While other triggers that contribute to muscular tension—they include negative emotional or mental states, such as stress, anxiety, and depression—can exacerbate the degree and frequency of headaches, these triggers cause pain *only* when combined with a weak and vulnerable structure. Because the single most determinant factor in biostructural vulnerability is poor posture, that is where we focus our attention for the remedy.

REMEDY: To eliminate the occurrence and recurrence of tension headaches, you need to have good posture, and good posture starts with good head position. The

TM addresses this concern by targeting the muscle groups that are intimately involved with facilitating posture and most responsible for causing tension headache symptoms. Specifically, it relaxes the muscles at the base of the skull (the suboccipital group) while tightening the muscles in the front of the neck. In the short term, the TM rapidly releases the overwhelming tension in the musculature of the region to bring about relief. In the long term, it corrects the misalignment of the head's position in relation to the spine. The TM also strengthens and balances the muscles needed to keep the head in optimal postural alignment. For additional long-term benefit you can add the Postural Correction TMs on page 190.

Note that this TM will prevent the onset of migraine or cluster headaches that are triggered by muscular tension.

Jaw (TMJ)

SYMPTOMS: Pain in the facial area and neck, headaches, limited movement in the jaw

INSTRUCTIONS: Open your mouth about an inch. Place your hand (palm down) underneath your chin and attempt to close the mouth by pressing upward (see 7–2). Resist the closing by keeping your jaw at the level of the original opening. Hold for six seconds. Close and relax the jaw. Do this motion five times for a total of 30 seconds. Repeat this TM daily until your symptoms are completely relieved.

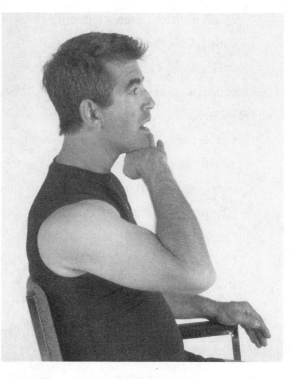

7–2. Jaw: Resistive Opening

CAUSE: You may not know this, but when you eat, speak, and yawn, you tend to the biological needs of your jaw. Like all other joints in the body, the jaw was made for movement. And like all other joints, it has to go through its full range of motion to maintain the optimal length of the muscles that serve it daily. For the most part, daily living provides for these needs. So, unlike most other joints in the body, the jaw does not require extra care to maintain its health. Under normal conditions it should function well for more than a century. Nonetheless, the jaw can fall prey to certain abnormalities and consequently it suffers erosion and arthritic changes, which makes even the simplest use painful. In the absence of dentistry problems, disease, and trauma, these abnormalities are a by-product of the musculoskeletal system.

When you have pain in the facial area, it is usually a warning sign that the temporomandibular joint of the jaw is in dysfunction. This disorder is more commonly known as TMJ. TMJ is a musculoskeletal condition that is often the direct result of the habitual clenching of the teeth. This clenching can be triggered unconsciously, through muscular imbalance or mental tension, or by a conscious act, such as chewing on a pen or biting the fingernails. Either way, the clenching causes a tightening of the muscle of mastication (chewing muscle) around the jaw joint. As the muscle clamps down on the jaw it inhibits its full range of motion, reduces the circulation to the area, and impedes frictionless movement, all of which cause localized pain. Because the muscle of mastication shares an intimate functional relationship with the muscles of the neck, its dysfunction can also contribute to headaches and neck pain. Eventually the constant clenching will cause the jaw to migrate and shift backward, further impeding normal function. Once the jaw adapts to this position, the cycle of clenching becomes ingrained in the musculature and will continue even in the absence of triggers.

REMEDY: TMJ can have serious consequences. Aside from the pain it causes, it can also limit two of the most basic human functions: eating and speaking. It is a progressive disorder but also a reversible one. To eradicate TMJ and relieve the resulting symptoms, the habitual cycle of clenching must be broken by patiently reeducating the musculature in the area. The TM accomplishes this by releasing tension and tightness from the muscles that close (or clench) the jaw while strengthening the oppositional muscles that open it. In the short term, the TM rapidly reduces your level of pain and clenching by relaxing the jaw and helping it to assume its appropriate position. In the long term, it fortifies and readapts the musculature toward normal placement. The TM also eliminates symptoms, corrects the inner mechanism of the jaw, and restores optimal function.

Note that if the pain in your jaw does not diminish in two to six weeks, you should consult a TMJ specialist.

Neck

SYMPTOMS: Stiffness; limited mobility; pain in the neck, face, or head

INSTRUCTIONS: While sitting or standing, bend your neck to the right as far as it can go so that your ear touches your left shoulder (see 7–3). Use your left hand to gently push your neck into that position. Keep your shoulders down throughout the motion. Hold for 30 seconds. Do the same motion to the left. Repeat this TM daily until your symptoms are completely relieved.

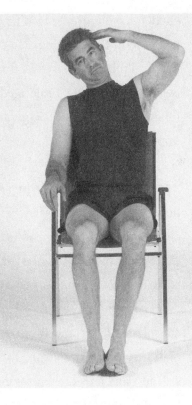

CAUSE: The neck is the connecting link between the base of the head and the top of the spine. Its precarious position and function in the body as both anchor and apex make it extremely vulnerable to both macrotraumatic and microtraumatic injuries.

7–3. Neck: Bends

Surprisingly, the biggest pain in the neck is not the result of things that happen during waking hours. That's right. Symptoms are usually the result of sleeping with improper spinal alignment. To sustain this poor sleeping position, the muscles in the neck have to continuously contract. On rising, the short, tight musculature manifests in a stiff and sore neck. Spending the next 8 to 10 hours in a static position—for instance, staring at a computer screen all day—compounds the dysfunction because it reinforces the reduced muscle length. This in turn overburdens and traumatizes the structure of the neck and the facet joints that connect the vertebrae in the region. Under these conditions, it isn't hard to see how just turning your head can cause so much pain.

Moreover, a pain in the neck is not, unfortunately, the only consequence of dysfunction in this region. The prolonged duress of abnormal forces due to short-ened musculature causes arthritis, deterioration of the structure, and limited movement. Dysfunction also contributes to the onset of headaches, facial discom-fort, and pinched nerves. A final consideration are the spinal discs sandwiched be-tween the vertebrae. Prolonged imposition can cause their premature dehydration, followed by actual breakage and nerve damage that brings pain to the neck and upper extremities.

REMEDY: After reading the preceding paragraphs, you probably want to run out to buy a new pillow. (See the Perfect Pillow Test on page 116 before you do.) While changing your sleeping habits will help to reduce the trauma to your neck, once you exhibit symptoms, only the total elimination of dysfunction will stop the recurring pain. To accomplish this, you must improve the mechanics of movement, restore op-timal posture, and stop the irritation to the tissues and discs. The TM addresses these considerations by stretching the muscles that are intimately involved with the motion of the neck while mobilizing the facet joints. In the short term, the TM rapidly relieves stiffness and tension by relaxing the musculature and improving circulation. It also takes the joints through their range of motion, thus promoting the necessary lubri-cation. In the long term, the TM eradicates dysfunction by balancing the musculature and restoring normal joint position and alignment. Most important, it promotes the ability to hold your head in its proper position, which is one of the fundamental building blocks of good posture and being pain free.

Shoulders

SYMPTOMS: Pain extending from the shoulder blade and running down the upper and lower arm, strain of the rotator cuff muscle, sprain, instability, limited movement, arthritis, tendonitis, bursitis, capsulitis

INSTRUCTIONS: Stand up and bend your elbows 90 degrees at waist height. Turn your hands palms up. Hold an exercise band (for less resistance, hold nothing) and pull it apart as far as you can while keeping your elbows next to your body (see 7–4a and 7–4b). Hold for six seconds and relax. Do this five times for a total of 30 seconds. Repeat this TM daily until your symptoms are completely relieved.

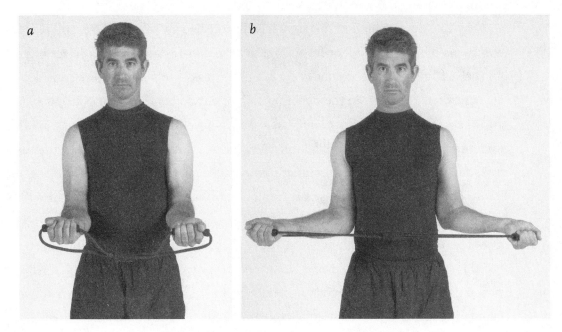

7–4a and b. Shoulders: Rotator Cuff Strengthener

Relief and Prevention for Less than a Buck

Exercise bands: $39.95

Rubber bands: 79¢ (for a whole bag)

It doesn't have to cost a lot to work. In fact, you can get the exact same benefits using cheap household rubber bands as you can from using expensive exercise bands. Just knot or tie the rubber bands together, making the length about a foot and a half. Proceed with the shoulder TM as instructed.

CAUSE: For thousands of years, we depended on the use of our upper extremities for survival. We climbed trees to forage for food, scaled mountains to survey the lay of the land, and threw rudimentary weapons to kill prey. As we came to rely more on tools and technology and less on our own physicality, our shoulders fell victim to much biomechanical dysfunction. Why? Because the biological needs of the joints and musculature in the shoulders were no longer met.

While the use of our shoulders has diminished substantially, we still place enormous demands on them from time to time. For instance, we reach up high on shelves, lift heavy objects above our heads, or play sports that require considerable exertion and agility in the upper portion of our bodies. We wear pocketbooks and knapsacks, carry briefcases and babies, and shovel snow and rake leaves. With undernourished joints and tight muscles, these mundane yet often strenuous tasks can produce both microtraumatic and macrotraumatic injuries.

The most common cause of shoulder pain is an injury to the rotator cuff muscles. The purpose of the rotator cuff muscles is twofold. First, they permit the movement of the arms both outward and inward. Second, they maintain the relationship between the two bones of the shoulder joints. You would think that with such big responsibilities, the rotators would be big muscles. In fact, they're not. Rotator cuff muscles are actually small and are highly prone to injury. Because their optimal length is rarely maintained, it doesn't take a lot to harm them. Just lifting a bag of groceries is sometimes enough to do the trick. Injured or dysfunctional rotator cuff muscles then cause irritation to the entire shoulder joint structure and increase friction during movement. This leads to many of the itises that we discussed earlier in the chapter, including arthritis, bursitis, capsulitis, and tendonitis.

REMEDY: It's hard to imagine that unloading the trunk of a car can cause so much trouble, but that's exactly what can happen if your shoulders are not in optimal condition. When there are symptoms of injury in the shoulder, you must correct the underlying dysfunction by challenging the muscles and joints within the limits of pain. The TM addresses this by targeting the range of motion of the shoulder joint and strengthening the rotator cuff muscles. In the short term, the TM rapidly initiates the healing process by strengthening the musculature while lubricating the entire shoulder joint capsule. In the long term, it brings about its complete healing by improving circulation in the region and stabilizing the shoulder joint. The TM also reduces the likelihood of future injuries to the rotator cuff.

Elbows

SYMPTOMS: Tennis elbow, severe pain and inflammation around the joint or both

INSTRUCTIONS: Make fists with both hands, tucking each thumb under the other four fingers. Place the back of your fists on a tabletop with the knuckles of the hands touching, and lean into the position so that your forearms are at 90-degree angles to your hands (see 7–5). Keep your elbows straight and locked throughout. Hold for 30 seconds. Repeat this TM daily until your symptoms are completely relieved.

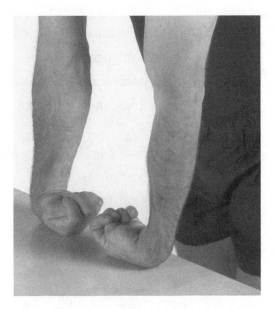

7–5. Elbows: Forearm Extensor Stretch

CAUSE: The elbow joint is quite stable and is not prone to the degree of arthritic changes found elsewhere in the body. Many in the medical establishment attribute its resilience to an innate physiological and genetic strength. I find no reason to believe this to be true. In fact, the health of the elbow is acquired. Because its full range of motion is consistently promoted through daily living and because as a result it is well lubricated with synovial fluid, the elbow's vulnerability to microtraumas is greatly diminished. This and this alone accounts for its remarkable ability to withstand constant wear and tear. However, the elbow is still susceptible to recurrent pain. If the biological needs of the elbow are so well served, is the joint the source of these disorders and its resulting pain? Or is there another culprit?

The forearm muscles that serve the elbow are an interesting and unusual group of muscles. They run more than half the entire length of the arm, starting just above the elbow and ending at the fingertips. They are unique in permitting movement of multiple joints. Thus, nearly all pain in the region—including pain in the elbows, wrists, hands, and fingers—is related to and caused by the forearm muscles. Specifically, pain in this region is a reliable indication that these muscles are not at their optimal lengths. Because the forearm muscles are strong, movement under the duress of their shortness and tightness imposes quite a bit of force on the multiple joints they serve. Although the elbow joint is structurally able to resist this imposition (the other joints are not), if the dysfunction persists and use continues under these conditions, local pain will occur.

REMEDY: You *can* play tennis without having to worry that you're going to pay a price for it later on. To relieve your symptoms and prevent their recurrence, you must restore the optimal lengths of your forearm muscles. I cannot overstate the importance of this. Functional and healthy forearm muscles benefit not only the elbow but every joint they serve. Thus the TM for the elbows also helps to relieve dysfunction of the wrists and their debilitating symptoms, such as carpel tunnel syndrome, and also dysfunction of the hands and fingers and the resulting symptoms, such as arthritic knuckles and trigger fingers.

This TM stretches part of the forearm muscle group by targeting the extensor muscles. In the short term, the TM rapidly relieves pain by releasing muscular tightness and tension. In the long term, it eliminates dysfunction in all the joints the forearm muscles serve.

Note that if you have pain, inflammation, or limited mobility in your wrists, hands, or fingers, include the elbow TM in your daily routine until your symptoms are completely gone.

Wrists

SYMPTOMS: Pain and inflammation in the wrist, arthritic changes, limited mobility, sprain

INSTRUCTIONS: Make a fist with your right hand. Bring your arm up to mid-torso height by bending your elbow 90 degrees. With your left hand, push your right wrist down toward the floor (see 7–6a). Resist the downward pushing for three seconds. Do this five times for a total of 15 seconds. Now, with your left hand, push your right wrist up toward the ceiling (see 7–6b). Resist the upward

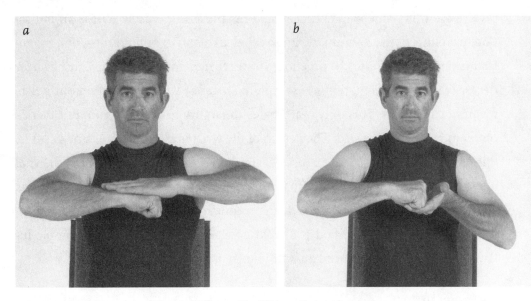

7–6a and b. Wrists: Strengthening

pushing. Do this five times for a total of 15 seconds. Switch hands. Repeat these TMs daily until your symptoms are completely relieved.

CAUSE: For those who don't have their wrists fixed in a contracted position all day—for instance, typing on a computer for eight hours—the health of the wrist is well maintained by a normal lifestyle. For the rest of us, the wrist is vulnerable to arthritic changes and pain. Here's why: The wrist is a relay station between the elbow and the hand. All three of these distinct regions share muscles that permit their movement: the forearm muscles. As you've just read, the forearm muscles are highly susceptible to dysfunction. When they are in dysfunction, every joint these short, tight muscles serve are adversely affected. While the elbow joint can withstand much of this muscular imposition, the wrist cannot. That's because the wrist is a highly complex joint, one in which eight bones (the carpals) come together instead of the usual two. To make matters worse, its biological needs—to be taken through its full range of motion daily—is rarely met. Any movement of this inherently vulnerable joint under conditions of insufficient lubrication, malnourishment, and muscular dysfunction can cause a whole assortment of ailments.

We are heavily dependent on the function of our wrists. Almost all activities involve them in some way. When symptoms present themselves, it is an indication that either a macrotraumatic injury, such as a sprain or tendinitis, or a microtraumatic injury, due to dysfunction, has occurred in the region. Out of sheer necessity we tend to ignore these symptoms because we are reliant on our wrists for most daily tasks. This only exacerbates the injury in the long run. But there's no room for such disregard. The design of the wrist is compact and, small as it is, filled with numerous bones, muscles, ligaments, and tendons. Moreover, vital nerves pass through it on their way from the arm to the hand. So minor problems are transformed into major ones. It isn't so much that the wrist suffers worse injuries than the rest of the body; it's that nowhere else in the body is simple inflammation more pronounced and more intrusive than in the wrist.

REMEDY: The wrist is infinitely complex, yet its restoration to optimal health is simple. One of the great anomalies of the wrist is that it is used constantly yet its musculature is often tight, weak, and imbalanced. To bring about relief and prevent further injuries, you need to strengthen and balance the musculature of the wrist. That is what the TMs do. They use upward and downward isometric resistance to strengthen the wrist. In the short term, the TMs rapidly stabilize the many joints in the region. In the long term, they bring about lasting relief, eliminate dysfunction, and build up tone, endurance, and resistance to repetitive use.

Wrists—Carpal Tunnel Syndrome (CTS)

SYMPTOMS: Tingling and numbness in the thumbs, pointers, and forefingers; pain, inflammation, and limited mobility in the wrists

EVALUATION: Before you treat carpal tunnel syndrome (CTS), you first need to establish whether you have it. Many people associate all pain in the wrists and hands with this condition, but CTS is only one of many possible causes of symptoms in this region. Here is a simple self-evaluation to help determine its likelihood: Raise both arms to chest height. Bend your elbows 90 degrees so that your hands are facing each other. From this starting position, bend your wrists 90 degrees, point your fingers to the floor, and press the back of your hands together so that you form the letter T with your arms and hands (see 7–7, page 168). Hold for 15 seconds. If you are able to do this motion without increasing your symptoms, it is likely that you do not have CTS. If this motion causes an increase in your symptoms, it is likely that you do have it. Proceed with the following TMs.

INSTRUCTIONS: The prescription for eradicating CTS is as follows: Repeat the elbow, wrist, and hands and fingers TMs daily until you are able to do the evaluation without pain or strain.

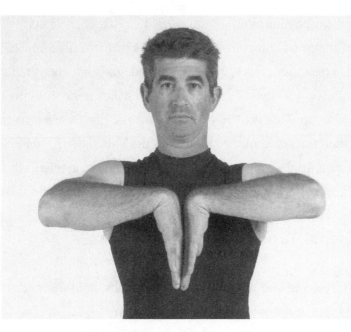

7–7. Carpal Tunnel Syndrome: Evaluation

CAUSE: CTS is one of the most common disorders of the wrist, so common that it's become part of our daily lexicon. Millions have been diagnosed with this condition, and the numbers are rising. It costs industry tens of millions of dollars in lost workdays and disability and leaves many people incapacitated, unemployed, and in pain. But it doesn't have to be this way. CTS is an acquired condition that can be relieved and, more important, prevented.

CTS, named after the narrow tunnel shaped by the carpal bones that make up the wrist, occurs when the joints, ligaments, tendons, and other structural components in the region become inflamed and impose on the limited space within the tunnel. Because the sensitive median nerve, which runs the length of the arm and into the hands and fingers, passes through the carpal tunnel, any swelling brings about tingling, numbness, pain, and, eventually, limited mobility. What causes the tissues in the wrist to swell? The prevailing theory is that repetitive movements, such as constant typing, irritate the tissue beyond its ability to function. In fact, repetitive movements will irritate tissue only if there is an underlying dysfunction there to begin with. Repetition and overuse have little or no effect on muscles that are strong, well balanced, and maintained at the proper length nor on joints that are fully lubricated with synovial fluid. However, even the most mundane tasks can cause significant injury to muscles that are weak, imbalanced, and shortened and to joints that are deprived of their synovial fluid. Demand plus neglect equals CTS.

REMEDY: Typing an e-mail doesn't have to be risky business. Your wrists have a long functional life span if they are properly cared for. To relieve symptoms, reverse CTS, and prevent its recurrence, you have to optimize the condition of all the muscles and joints that affect the performance of the wrist. Because the wrist is intimately connected to the elbow, hand, and fingers, you must do all of the corresponding TMs until symptoms of CTS are completely gone.

Hands and Fingers

SYMPTOMS: Pain in the knuckles and palms, inflammation of the region's tendons and joints, limited movement of the fingers

INSTRUCTIONS: Extend your hands in front of you at chest height with the fingers of each hand touching. Quickly spread them apart so that you feel a stretch (see 7–8), then close them as hard as you can back to the starting position. Do this 15 times. Repeat this TM daily until your symptoms are completely relieved.

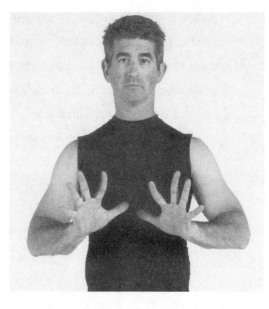

CAUSE: Nearly all of the intricate and complex endeavors imagined by the human mind are carried through to fruition by the hands and fingers. They are the anatomical well from which most achievement springs.

7–8. Hands and Fingers: Strengthener

Because the hands and fingers play a constant role in almost all activity, the everyday biological needs of the joints in this region are well served. Nonetheless, their primary movements—specifically, opening and closing—are often done under the duress of the short, tight musculature of the forearms. Dysfunction of the forearm muscles causes many problems to the hands and fingers. They include arthritic knuckles, limited mobility, and pain.

While the forearm muscles are responsible for a good portion of the problems in this region, the intrinsic muscles of the hands are also prone to dysfunction. These muscles make it possible to bring your fingers closer together and spread them farther apart. When they are dysfunctional, even the simplest of tasks can be impossible to carry out. Because the TMs for the elbows and wrists address the forearm muscles that move the fingers, we turn our attention to the intrinsic musculature for remedying of hand and finger dysfunction.

REMEDY: When you exhibit symptoms in your hands and fingers, it is an indication that arthritic changes may already have taken place in the region. I've seen many patients who, because of the crippling consequences of arthritis, cannot even button their shirt or sign their name. It greatly saddens me because arthritis that is not related to disease is an acquired pathology. To stop its further progression, you must eliminate the dysfunction in the region's musculature. This TM strengthens and stretches the intrinsic muscles. In the short term, the TM rapidly brings blood and healing nutrients into the area while removing excessive inflammatory fluid. In the long term, the TM relieves symptoms and halts the progression of further arthritic changes. Even more significant, it restores optimal health to the hands and fingers, which helps to overcome changes that may have already occurred.

Note that your hands and fingers will benefit significantly by including the elbow and wrist TMs in your daily routine until symptoms are gone.

Upper Back

SYMPTOMS: Discomfort or pain in the region, muscle spasms along the upper back, limited movement

INSTRUCTIONS: Sit in a chair with an immobile upright backrest. Elevate your arms over your head and place one hand in the palm of the other. Lean backward six inches, letting your head follow the lead of your arms (see 7–9). Hold the position for 30 seconds. Repeat this TM daily until your symptoms are completely relieved.

CAUSE: When a person says that his or her "back is out," he or she is usually referring to the lower back. And indeed, the upper back is generally free of the devastating effects of pain. Why is this so? Gross movement of the spine occurs mostly in the lower back and the neck. Thus the upper back is spared the macro-

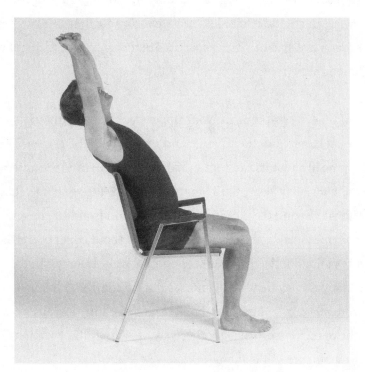

7–9. Upper Back: Stretch

traumatic and microtraumatic consequences of large movements. The upper back also has the added protection of the rib cage. The rib cage, as its name implies, acts to secure the contents it encloses. It limits the amount of spinal deviation in the upper back and helps stabilize the facet joints in the region. But there is a downside. Every rib is attached to the spine with two joints instead of the usual one. This makes them more vulnerable than other joints in the body. Fortunately, these joints aren't subjected to much movement. Unfortunately, they are highly vulnerable to one of the hallmarks of modern culture: poor posture.

When you have pain or, more commonly, discomfort in your upper back, it is a sign that poor posture has caused the joints of the upper spine to become misaligned. How does this happen? The facet joints of the spine are like oval tea plates. Under optimal postural conditions, these plates stack perfectly one on top of another. Poor standing, sitting, and sleeping postures cause the joints to shift slightly out of their proper position. To accommodate this small deviation, the musculature reacts by contracting. Eventually the joints settle out of alignment, and the muscles, in an effort to shield the area from further injury, go into what's known as a protective spasm. These spasms are the source of pain, inflammation, and dysfunction in the region.

REMEDY: To relieve symptoms in your upper back and maintain its long-lasting health, you must target both the rib cage and vertebrae in the region. The TM takes the thoracic spine through its range of motion while stretching the anterior muscles of this region. In the short term, the TM rapidly realigns the vertebrae, fully lubricates the joints with vital synovial fluid, and releases tension from the musculature, all of which reduce symptoms. In the long term, it brings about better overall posture, stabilization of the joints, and a restoration of optimal muscle length in the upper back.

Note that you may hear bodily noises during the TM. If you do, don't worry. It's the sound of your upper back being cracked—terminology you may have heard in a chiropractor's office—another way of saying that your joints are being put back into their correct positions.

Lower Back

SYMPTOMS: Localized pain, spasms, limited mobility, inability to function

EVALUATION: Before you begin the lower-back TM, you should establish whether a herniated disc is the cause of your symptoms. Here is a simple self-evaluation to help determine if this is so: Sit on a chair and slowly bend over so that your hands interlace behind your calves (see 7–10). If you are able to do this without increasing your symptoms, it is likely that you do not have a herniated disc. Proceed with the following TM. If this motion causes an increase in your symptoms—at which point you should stop immediately—you may have a herniated disc. Do *not* proceed with the following TM until you consult a health care professional for further evaluation.

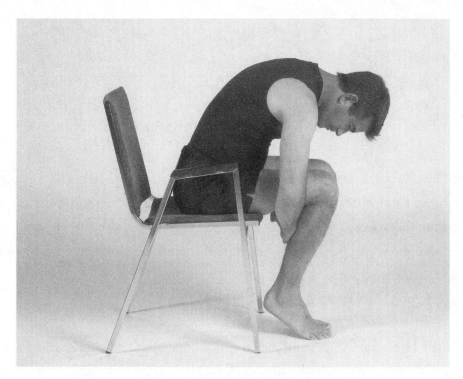

7–10. Herniated Disc: Evaluation

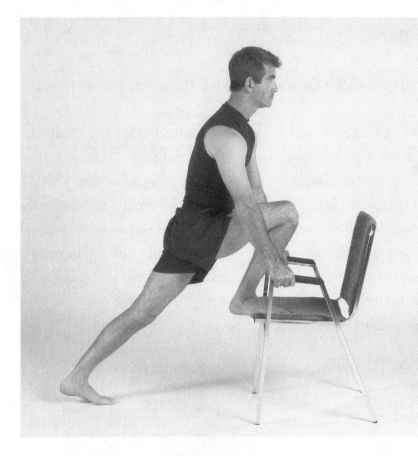

7–11. Lower Back: Hip Flexor Stretch

INSTRUCTIONS: Stand up and place your right foot on a chair, table, or stair that is two to three feet high. Step back approximately three feet with your left leg and point that foot straight ahead. Gently lean forward until you feel a stretch in your outer groin area (see 7–11). Your left heel should come off the ground as you lunge. Hold for 30 seconds. Switch legs. Repeat this TM daily until your symptoms are completely relieved.

CAUSE: More than 80 percent of the global population will suffer at least one episode of severe lower-back pain in their lives. Most will suffer chronically. Lower-back pain is the one reason why people go to doctors, take medications, and miss work. It is also one of the most common and costly medical problems in the world. What makes the lower back prone to so much misery? Truth be told, it's a very long story. Here's the short version.

Let me start by saying that there isn't anything inherently wrong with the lower back. Its structural design is flawless. It is made up of sturdy anatomical elements that include muscles, ligaments, tendons, and five bony vertebrae and the protective cushiony discs they sandwich. The lower back is located near the center of gravity, making it the functional Grand Central Terminal of the body. What are the ramifications of this? The lower back has to accommodate all of the functions both above and below it. Under optimal total body conditions, this would have little effect. Under less than optimal conditions, such as poor head and neck posture, rounded shoulders, upper spinal misalignment, weak abdominal muscles, dysfunctional hips, unstable knees, and injured ankles, the consequences to the lower back are catastrophic. Moreover, the area has to contend with its own weak, imbalanced musculature, underlubricated facet joints, and discs that are susceptible to herniation and rupture. Any one of the items on this long list is enough to cause problems in the region. The reality is that most people suffer from some, if not all, of the dysfunctions listed above. And then they wonder how they threw their backs out again.

REMEDY: If any one region benefits most from the total body approach of the 3-Minute Maintenance Method, it is the lower back. You simply cannot avoid lower-back pain without addressing the totality of your being. That said, there are targeted and focused ways to reduce some of the common weaknesses of the lower back while increasing some of its strengths. The TM stretches the hip flexors, the muscles responsible for much dysfunction in the region. In the short term, the TM rapidly eliminates dysfunction and reduces the stress to the lumbar spine, which lessens the burden on the lower back. In the long term, it brings about lasting relief by balancing the structure and the whole region. The TM also makes the lower back far less susceptible to injury and pain by reducing the stress from the enormous demands placed on it.

Lower Back—Sciatica

SYMPTOMS: Shooting pain or tingling down the length of the leg (or both), often in conjunction with limited mobility and lower-back pain

EVALUATION: Before you treat sciatica, you need to know whether or not the sciatic nerve is irritated by the spinal discs or by the piriformis muscle. Here is a simple self-evaluation to help determine which is the case: Lie flat on your back on the floor. Lift your head and shoulders off the ground and look at your toes. Without bending your knee, slowly lift your right leg off the ground approximately three feet or 30 degrees (see 7–12). If this motion causes an increase in your symptoms, your sciatica is probably disc related and you should consult with a health care professional. If you can do this motion without increasing your symptoms, your sciatica is probably muscular. Proceed with the following TM.

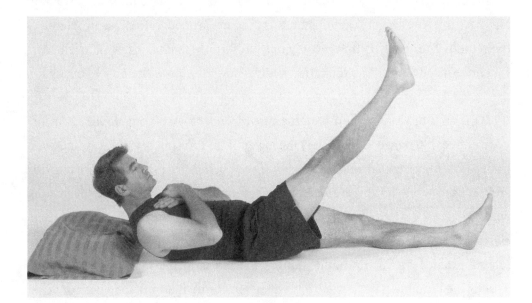

7–12. Sciatica: Evaluation

INSTRUCTIONS: Sit on a chair and place your right ankle on your left knee. Grab hold of your right knee with both hands and bring it up and across your body toward your left shoulder so that your thigh touches your chest (see 7–13). Hold for 30 seconds. Switch legs. Repeat this TM daily until your symptoms are completely relieved.

CAUSE: Sciatica is a painful, often debilitating condition, unsurprisingly so since it occurs when the largest nerve in the body becomes inflamed. What causes the inflammation to occur? The sciatic is a long cablelike nerve approximately the thickness of your pinky. It has its roots in the lower back, runs down the entire length of your leg, and ends at your toes. The sciatic nerve is unfortunately located

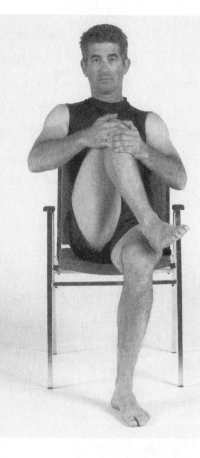

7–13. Sciatica: Piriformis Stretch

in some of the body's most vulnerable regions. This, coupled with its size, makes it ripe for irritation. On the nerve's large, vulnerable surface area are two hot spots that cause the majority of its irritation: the lower back and the hips.

    The lower back is made up of bony vertebrae that sandwich protective gel-like cushions called discs. These discs are highly sensitive and are especially susceptible to wear and tear. Because the lower back is one of the most used, abused, and neglected areas of the body, the discs there often bulge or herniate under the constant pressure. If the herniation occurs near the sciatic nerve, it presses on its roots. The nerve responds to this imposition, producing referred pain down the back of the leg.

The hip region, another of the most used, abused, and neglected areas of the body, houses a muscle called the piriformis. When the hips fall prey to dysfunction, strain, and injury, the piriformis begins to tighten, and eventually goes into spasm. Unfortunately, the sciatic nerve passes underneath, sometimes directly through, the piriformis muscle on its way down the leg. The spasmodic muscle traps and compresses the sciatic nerve, which can cause symptoms anywhere from your buttocks to the tips of your toes.

REMEDY: Once you have evaluated your condition and determined that the sciatic nerve is irritated by the piriformis muscle, you need to take the pressure off the nerve. The TM stretches the piriformis muscle and the other muscles in the area. In the short term, the TM rapidly helps to reduce the pressure on the sciatic nerve by relaxing the piriformis muscle. As the pressure on the nerve subsides, so too will your symptoms. In the long term, the TM maintains the optimal length of the piriformis, making it less likely to go into spasm as a result of other dysfunction in the region.

Hips

SYMPTOMS: Pain in the hips and pelvic girdle, muscle spasms, limited mobility, arthritis, bursitis

INSTRUCTIONS: Sit with your buttocks on the edge of a chair. Extend your legs so that your knees are straight and your heels touch the floor. Place your heels two feet apart. Roll your legs outward so that the outsides of your feet touch the floor (see 7–14a), then roll them inward so that the insides of your feet touch the ground (see 7–14b). Slowly roll back and forth 15 times for a total of 30 seconds. Repeat this TM daily until your symptoms are completely relieved.

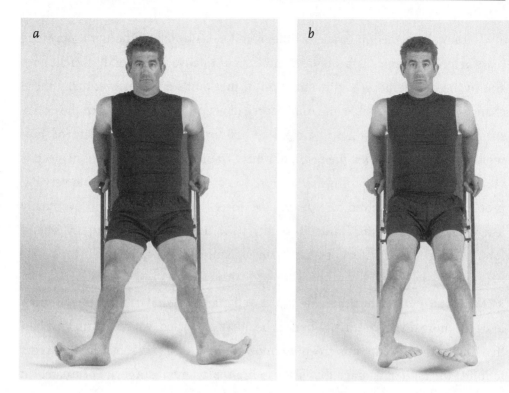

7–14a and b. Hips: Rolls

CAUSE: The hip is a strong, sturdy, and stable joint. It is well constructed and is nestled safely in a region of the body that protects it from injury. It is well suited to its task and is well engineered to permit the type of movement it was made for. Then why on earth do tens of millions of people around the world need hip-replacement surgery, making it the number two most common joint replacement surgery each year?

The hip is in trouble because of how it's treated. Quite simply, the hip is used and abused more than almost any other joint in the body. Its biological needs are severely underserved in that the hip is rarely taken through its full range of motion and the muscles that serve it are rarely maintained at their optimal length. At the same time, the demands placed on it are enormous. The hip carries the bulk of the body's weight, is subjected to the pull of the most powerful muscles in the body, and is under almost constant pressure. Most important, the debilitating consequences of prolonged sitting most significantly affect the hip. The sum total of this dysfunction is catastrophic.

Damage to the hip happens little by little, day by day. Although it may take years before symptoms appear, the silent but cumulative effects of dysfunction result in the deterioration and destruction of the joint's surface. Eventually these changes will be irreversible; the only course of action then is to replace the entire structure. It is interesting to note that the overwhelming majority of hip-replacement surgery is *not* the result of injury, trauma, or disease but of neglect. If you have recurrent symptoms in your hip, you are already on the road to very big problems. Left unresolved, the destructive forces of dysfunction will eventually lead to crippling arthritis, limited mobility, pain, medication, and surgery. Therefore, it is imperative that you be especially vigilant with the care of your hips.

REMEDY: When the health of the hip is well maintained, it can last free of problems for more than a century. When its health is neglected, you won't make it half that time without symptoms creeping into your life. As stated above, it takes years to inflict the kind of damage that leads to hip-replacement surgery. Fortunately, it doesn't take years to repair. Indeed, eliminating the cause of dysfunction stops the irritation to the joint almost instantaneously. The TM mobilizes the hip, causing the joint to be lubricated with synovial fluid. In the short term, the TM rapidly increases movement and flexibility by relaxing muscular tightness. In the long term, it brings about lasting relief to the hip and the lower back, makes the hip less vulnerable to injury and dysfunction, and heals some of the structural damage incurred during the years of use and abuse.

Knees

SYMPTOMS: Pain, inflammation, spasms, limited mobility, sprains, strains, arthritis, bursitis, synovitis, tendinitis

INSTRUCTIONS: Sit on a chair and lift both feet about two inches off the floor. Cross your right ankle over your left and press it against the left ankle as hard as

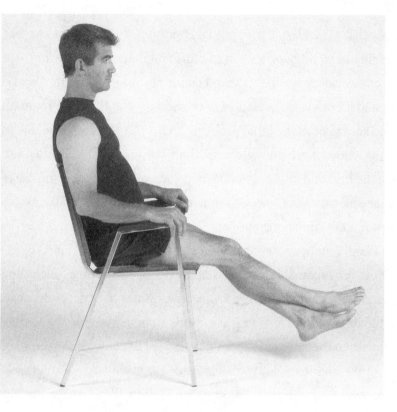

7–15. Knees: Strengthener

you can (see 7–15). Resist the downward push for five seconds. Relax and switch feet. Do the entire procedure six times for a total of 30 seconds per leg. Repeat this TM daily until your symptoms are completely relieved.

CAUSE: The most commonly performed joint-replacement surgeries are knee and hip, respectively. The hip is a stable joint; the knee is not. The knee is the largest and most complex joint in the body and also one of the most vulnerable. It is situated between the two long bones of the leg, so the forces that act on it—from above and below—are considerable. It is a complicated structure that permits mobility without the security of sturdy encapsulation. In other words, the knee is designed to favor flexible movement at the expense of remaining intact. On top of that, we walk a lot, go up and down stairs, sprint across streets, and engage in sports and recreation, all with knees that are in less than optimal condition. Is it any wonder that they are highly prone to a plethora of microtraumatic and macrotraumatic injuries?

The knee joint operates at a mechanical disadvantage that makes it even more dependent on its musculature to provide its stability and proper alignment. This is the source of many of its problems. The knee is like the elbow in that the muscles that move it, which include the hamstrings and quadriceps, serve multiple joints: the hips and knees. Because large demands are placed on these muscles and because normal lifestyle does not promote their optimal length, they are highly prone to dysfunction. The knee is structurally less sound than the sturdy elbow and is ill equipped to handle the imposition of these short, tight muscles. Dysfunction is responsible for a wide range of symptoms, including muscle strain, tears, spasms, and rupture. It also contributes to sprains, dislocations, and many of the itises we discussed earlier in this chapter. And the problems don't end there. Injuries to the knee cause varying degrees of changes to your gait, and any variation in the alignment of your legs and feet inhibits your ability to maintain optimal posture. Furthermore, the knee is functionally related to the hips, pelvis, upper and lower legs, ankles, and feet. Because it is the midpoint in this anatomical chain, injuries to the knee affect all of these areas as well.

REMEDY: The knee is prone to injury, but it isn't fragile. Its susceptibility is a direct result of neglect, which is exacerbated by the amount and type of use we put it through every day. To relieve symptoms and protect the knee from reinjury, you need to build up the endurance of the musculature and eliminate knee dysfunction. The TM addresses this by strengthening the hamstrings and quadriceps equally. In the short term, the TM rapidly tones and balances the musculature, making activities easier and less risky, and initiates the healing process. In the long term, it progressively builds strength to create a stable knee, restores normal function to the region, and reduces the knee's vulnerability to injury.

Shin Splints

SYMPTOMS: Pain between knee and ankle; tangible herniation, bulging, or superficial inflammation in the area of the shin

INSTRUCTIONS: Take off your shoes. Kneel on the floor so that the tops of your feet touch it and gently sit back on your heels (see 7–16). Hold for 30 seconds. Repeat this TM daily until your symptoms are completely relieved and always before a workout.

CAUSE: At some point in your life, you will probably attempt to exercise. The likelihood is that you will do so without knowing whether your body is prepared for the chosen activity. One of the ramifications of overexerting or overextending a dysfunctional body is shin splints. Shin splints are one of

7–16. Shin Splints: Long Muscle Stretch

the few musculoskeletal disorders that are a direct result of exercise, not general use. If you've ever taken up jogging, you've probably experienced shin splints. Although shin splints may seem to be nothing more than an interruptive nuisance at the time, they can have some surprising consequences.

There are very few muscles in the body whose health you can ignore without paying a price. The muscle in your shin is one of them. For the most part, you would not know it was there if it weren't for those—dare I say, rare—times when you venture out for a cardiovascular workout. Piercing and sharp pain in your shin reminds you that in fact a muscle is at work there; specifically, a hardworking, short, and tight muscle. A shin splint occurs when the connective tissue that covers the shin muscle is subjected to powerful forces, such as running, jumping, and brisk walking, that it cannot handle in its dysfunctional state. The connective tissue tears, and the shin muscle eventually herniates or bulges, which produces the pain you feel. Gentle pressure on the shin at the moment the splint occurs is highly effective at relieving the pain, but it is only a temporary solution because the underlying dysfunction has not been addressed. That is why shin splints have a high rate of recurrence. If the dysfunction remains unresolved and overuse continues, the tissue will deteriorate. Eventually the chronic disorder will inhibit your ability to participate in demanding physical activity.

REMEDY: With all the things that can go wrong with the musculoskeletal system, who wants to bother with the shins? Well, if you exercise and want to keep engaging in cardiovascular activity, it is imperative that you pay attention to the health of the musculature there. Failure to do so ensures that shin splints will continue to plague your workouts, not only causing excruciating pain but also interfering with your ability to participate in other exercise regimens. To therapeutically relieve your symptoms, you must restore the optimal length of the shin muscle. The TM stretches the muscle in the region. In the short term, this TM should relieve your pain completely. However, the absence of symptoms doesn't mean that you should no longer include this TM in your daily routine. In the long term, its daily application increases the stamina of the shin muscle, which reduces the likelihood of any recurrence. If you are prone to shin splints, you should continue to do this TM before every cardiovascular workout.

Ankles

SYMPTOMS: Pain, swelling, inflammation, and limited mobility or function at the ankle; tendonitis; synovitis; sprain

INSTRUCTIONS: Place a workout step in front of you. It should be from two to four inches in height. Place the top half of both feet (up to the balls of your feet) on the step while keeping the heels on the ground (see 7–17). Lean your weight into it, making sure that your posture remains straight. You should feel the stretch in your ankle and calf muscles. Hold for 30 seconds. Repeat this TM daily until your symptoms are completely relieved.

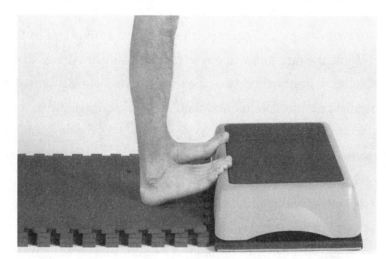

7–17. Ankles: Achilles Stretch

Relief and Prevention for Less than a Buck

Workout step: **$49.95**

Toilet paper: **pennies per roll**

You can get the exact same benefits using rolls of toilet paper as you can from using an expensive workout step! Place two rolls (make sure they're full ones, double-padded recommended) on the floor and proceed with the ankles TM as instructed.

CAUSE: Ankles are under a lot of pressure: Even when you're just standing still, nearly 100 percent of the body's weight bears down on them. Now imagine what happens to your weight distribution when you lift up one leg. The weight that was equally distributed is now loaded completely on one ankle. Put that leg down and lift the other and the weight transfers completely to the other ankle. The net effect—which, by the way, is what happens when you walk—is that the force per ankle doubles. Increase the rate at which you lift each leg—in jogging, for example—and the force quadruples. Run and that number doubles. You get the picture. Under these conditions, it seems miraculous that ankles last at all. But they do. Ankles are sturdy joints and are well designed to carry out the job they were intended for, namely, locomotion. While they are prone to microtraumatic injuries due to dysfunctional muscles and joints, it is more likely that the pain you are feeling is caused by macro-traumatic injuries, such as sprains, and their residual consequences.

Every joint in the human body has receptors in its capsules and ligaments. These receptors send signals to the brain so that it can monitor changes in position. This vital mechanism permits the body to react and adjust quickly and appropriately to the constant shift of bodily movement. When a joint is injured, its receptors are damaged. Although the injury may heal, these damaged receptors never regenerate. Thus the feedback from the joint to the brain is reduced, and permanent deficiency at the site of the injury is created. Most joints can withstand this reduction of receptors because they are not prone to macrotraumatic injuries. This is not so with the ankle joints. The ankles are more prone to macrotraumatic injuries, such as sprains and strains from tripping, twisting, and misstepping, than any other joint in the body. Without the full availability of the feedback mechanism, the ankles are under the constant threat of further traumas. This has a profound effect on the anatomy. Not only does the ankle lose its stability but further injuries also leave residual scars in its tissues, which limits its function. This scar tissue weakens the ankle and causes additional dysfunction. In turn, the dysfunction causes more injury. It is a viscious, self-perpetuating cycle that inevitably leads to pain, arthritis, and limited mobility.

REMEDY: Twisting your ankle or stepping awkwardly off a curb are events that happen all the time. So it's inevitable that you're going to lose some receptors in your ankle joints. But this doesn't mean that you have to lose the full function of your ankles. In fact, you can relieve your symptoms and protect your ankles from further harm. The TM takes the ankles through their range of motion and stretches the Achilles tendon. In the short term, the TM rapidly relieves symptoms by reducing inflammation in the tendon. In the long term, it helps to balance the entire ankle structure. The TM also restores the O.M.L. of the muscle groups that govern movement at the ankle, causing them to become a better feedback mechanism. Muscles that are rehabilitated in this fashion become so well tuned to reactive motion that they compensate for some loss of receptors in the ankle joints.

Note that an additional way to enhance the receptors in your ankle joints is to balance on each foot for 30 seconds daily.

Feet and Toes

SYMPTOMS: Pain in the feet, toes, or both; limited mobility or function of the toes; fatigue; cramping

INSTRUCTIONS: Take off your shoes. Kneel and place the pads of your toes on the floor. Sit back on your heels gently so that your toes bend backward about an inch (see 7–18). Hold for 30 seconds. Repeat this TM daily until your symptoms are completely relieved.

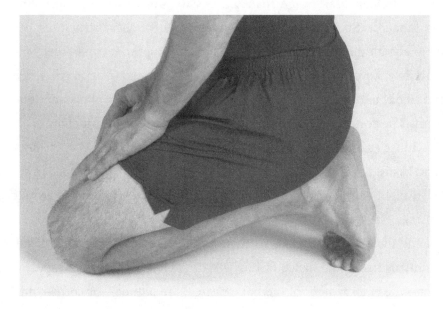

7–18. Feet and Toes: Stretch

CAUSE: Believe it or not, cavemen didn't wear Nikes. In fact, for thousands of years, humankind walked around barefoot. Without even knowing it, Fred and Wilma Flintstone benefited by meeting the biological needs of their feet and toes daily. How? Natural terrain varies considerably, not only over large expanses of land but step by step. To accommodate these variations, the feet and toes had to be flexible enough to instantaneously and continuously adapt and adjust. The conditions of constantly walking barefoot allowed our ancestors' joints to go through their full range of motion and the muscles to maintain their optimal length.

Then along came the shoe. Shoes are a wonderful invention. They protect the soles of the feet from injuries incurred when stepping on difficult terrain and sharp objects and from dangerous animals. But there is a trade-off. What we gain in protection we lose in the full movement of our feet and toes. And that deficiency is responsible for the pain you feel in this region.

Feet ground you to . . . the ground. They are the base of your body, and their marvelous architectural design makes it possible for them to perform their intended function. Specifically, they are made up of arches, structures perfectly suited to absorb the impact of heavy loads. Under optimal conditions, your feet should rarely if ever be a source of symptoms or fatigue. However, after prancing around all day under the unnatural subjugation of shoes, it's no wonder that your feet hurt. The restrictive nature of shoes causes painful dysfunction in the numerous muscles and joints of the region. The restriction also causes the foot to step flat. Instead of falling squarely on the arch—which is able to sustain the load of body weight—the force of stepping is directed upward and onto areas of the musculoskeletal system that are unable to cope with the additional pressure. Finally, some shoes, especially those with a high heel, cause the pressure of stepping to continually fall on the instep or the balls of the feet. This leads, respectively, to bunions—the enlargement of the bone nearest the big toe—or corns—the hardening of the skin due to improper friction—both extremely painful disorders.

Shoes, however, are here to stay. In the world we live in, it would be impractical even to think about not wearing them. Because most of us experience pain in our feet and toes from time to time, we go to some lengths to help the situation. For instance, some people wear only expensive ergonomic shoes. Much like expensive ergonomic chairs, these shoes make a bad situation a little better but still contribute to dysfunction since they're still shoes. Some think that walking around barefoot for a small portion of the day will do the trick. They should think again. Going around barefoot in the park, house, or even the shower actually exacerbates dysfunction and increases wear and tear because the muscles and joints in the region are no longer adaptable. Still others soak their feet in hot water or treat them to a massage now and then. These practices do relieve symptoms, but they are only temporary solutions. Is there any way to protect and preserve the anatomy that quite literally walks us through our lives? You bet there is.

REMEDY: Your poor aching feet are screaming for attention. The way to protect them from the consequences of wearing shoes is to optimize the health of the muscles and joints in the region. And there are lots of them. Indeed, the function of the feet and toes is infinitely complex. However, tending to their biological needs is actually quite simple. The TM targets the toe joints by taking them through their range of motion while stretching the musculature in the region. In the short term, the TM rapidly relieves cramping, fatigue, pain, and inflammation. In the long term, it allows the joints to be fully lubricated and restores the optimal length of the muscles, thus preventing arthritis and limited function. The TM also helps to prevent bunions and corns by reducing stress to the susceptible areas.

Poor Posture

SYMPTOMS: Rounded shoulders; acquired postural deviations, such as rounded back (hyperkyphosis); headaches; neck and back pain; fatigue; depression; shortness of breath; limitation of bodily function

INSTRUCTIONS: Stand in a doorway with your feet shoulder-width apart. Place your toes just inside the line of the frame and lift your arms so that the palms of your hands touch the top of the doorway. Keep your arms and palms shoulder-width apart. Tighten your stomach muscles and squeeze your buttocks together. From this starting position, lean forward approximately one to two feet (see 7–19). Be sure to keep your head in alignment with your back. Hold for 30 seconds. Next, sit in a chair. Without exaggerating your posture, try to replicate a good standing posture by keeping your back straight, shoulders back, and chin parallel to the floor. Put your arms behind your head and clasp your palms together. Open your elbows as far as you can while pushing back against your palms with your head (see 7–20). Hold for 30 seconds. Repeat both of these TMs daily until you see noticeable improvement in both your standing and seated posture.

CAUSE: We have all been pestered at some point in our lives to "stand up straight." This is mostly for aesthetic reasons. It simply does not look good to slouch. But the ramifications of poor posture go way beyond anything that can be seen with the naked eye. Poor posture—the improper alignment of the spine—affects the health of the entire body, including almost all muscles, joints, and vital organs. It also affects the ability to breathe correctly, think clearly, and function without incurring the plethora of chronic ailments that abound today.

Evolution formed the human organism both to stand erect and withstand the constant force of gravity. The spinal column, which runs down the center of the human body, is the structure that makes this possible (see Chapter 3, page 64, for more on the spine). Its characteristic S curve is a perfected design that is maintained by the posture we keep when walking, standing, and sitting. If the shape of

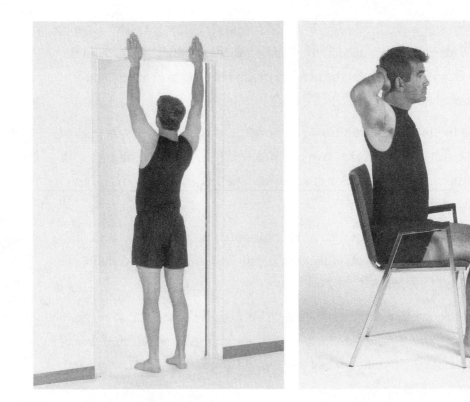

7–19. *Postural Correction: Standing*   7–20. *Postural Correction: Seated*

this curve is maintained, the spine is able to provide the agility to interact with the environment in a flexible way while distributing the stress of movement and gravity to the anatomy most capable of handling them. If the shape of the curve is not maintained, the opposite occurs. The agility and flexibility of the spine are inhibited and the stress of movement and gravity are distributed to parts of the anatomy less capable of handling them. The consequences are devastating. You would think that with so much at stake maintaining optimal posture would be a top priority. In fact, I have met very few people in my life whose posture even comes close to optimal.

Poor posture is caused by poor choices. While some postural deviations are inherited, such as some forms of scoliosis, or are brought on by trauma, such as a car accident, the vast majority of postural abnormalities are caused by things within our sphere of control:

- We live in a physically deprived and sedentary culture, which creates a weakness in our musculature. Weak muscles are unable to expend the energy needed to hold the head, neck, and back in proper position throughout the day.

- We live in a sitting culture that spends inordinately long hours in chairs. The seated position is at best an unnatural one. At worst, sitting compromises the relationship between the spine and pelvic region, including the hips.

- We are an overweight society. Excessive body weight throws muscular balance completely off kilter, thus greatly imposing on the vertebrae and joints of the spine.

- We are an often depressed people. This negative emotional state produces a protective slouch. And vice versa: Slouching reduces self-confidence, increases the number of bad moods, and adversely affects our general sense of well-being.

- We are unaware of what proper posture is and choose not to spend our time learning how to properly cultivate it.

While this may seem to be an insurmountable list, the good news is that these are all acquired habits. And habits, after all, are made to be broken.

REMEDY: Optimal posture is an achievable goal. For some, the years of slouching and slumping may have taken their toll to such an extent that the disfigurement to the spine can be corrected only with specialized equipment. For most people, how-ever, the restoration of normal posture can be made with a few simple adjustments. To bring about optimal posture, the head should be maintained at a level horizontal position, the spine should maintain its S curvature, and the legs should maintain a straight line to the floor. These three principles are based on standing posture. The same principles apply to the seated posture. Both TMs address these considerations

Relief and Prevention for Less Than a Buck

Ergonomic chair: $800 to $2,000

Roll of paper towels: 99¢

It is almost impossible to maintain optimal posture while sitting. That is why it's is so bad for you, no matter how cheap or expensive the chair you sit in. However, lumbar support can help some. You can save big bucks by using an ordinary paper towel roll to provide the same benefits. Just place it in the space between your lower back and the chair and adjust it (by removing towels) so that it exactly fills the gap. Once it's the right size, take a string and thread it through the roll and around the chair. Tie a secure knot. Replace the roll when the paper towels wear down.

but from different angles. The first TM stretches the entirety of the spinal musculature. The second TM stretches the musculature in the neck, shoulders, and upper back. In the short term, the TMs rapidly rebalance the muscles and realign the spinal vertebrae. They also strengthen the muscles most intimately involved with proper head and neck posture. In the long term, the TMs maintain the proper curvature of the spine; strengthen the pelvic and abdominal muscles, which play an intimate role in optimal posture; and lubricate the spinal facet joints. They also promote upper-spinal alignment and optimal postural maintenance.

The keys to the success of the TMs in this chapter are consistent daily application and continuation even after symptoms subside. The longer you do double duty by including them in your daily routine, the more pronounced the long-term benefits will be.

At the first sign of pain, do not hesitate to return to this chapter for rapid relief and healing. It is hoped that the 3-Minute Maintenance Method and the 3-Month Tune-Up will keep you away from these pages. But if you're ever in need, the TMs in this chapter are here to help.

Happy Endings: Sheldon's Story

Sheldon R., age 61, is a successful ophthalmic surgeon, an aspiring golfer, and an avid wine connoisseur. He is also among the millions of people who have suffered from an assortment of chronic musculoskeletal pain for much of their lives. We have been friends for almost two decades, although we met under inauspicious circumstances.

Sixteen years ago I bought one of those compact cars that are good for the environment. Unfortunately, the contour of the driver's seat in this particular car wasn't so good for my back. But I didn't know that at the time. After driving around in it for a few weeks, I developed an ache in my lower back. One afternoon shortly thereafter, I drove with my wife to a party. When we arrived, I had a massive muscle spasm that pinched my sciatic nerve. The horrific pain left me unable to exit the car. I asked my wife to go into the party to see if there was a doctor in the house. That's how I met Dr. Joseph Weisberg.

To treat the sciatic crisis, Dr. Weisberg immediately iced my back for 20 minutes, then gently guided me through some of his therapeutic movements (TMs). While this treatment gave me some instantaneous relief, he explained that a full recovery required a continuation of his targeted TMs for an additional two to six weeks. As prescribed, I employed his TMs daily for the next month, even though my symptoms had abated in the first 72 hours. Because I periodically add the sciatic TMs to his daily maintenance program to this day, I have managed to avoid sciatic flare-ups ever since. By the way, I also got rid of the car.

As a medical professional, I am very familiar with the modalities used to treat musculoskeletal pain and know of no other that is as effective—both for short-term relief and long-term restoration to function—as Dr. Weisberg's methodology. His TMs not only rapidly relieve the sensation of pain, they also eradicate the underlying condition that triggered the onset of pain in the first place. This is a vital distinction because in treating the cause, not just the effects of musculoskeletal dysfunction, true healing is likely to occur. This is in stark contrast to many traditional medical treatments, such as medications and surgery, which reduce the effects but often not the cause of musculoskeletal dysfunction. Dr. Weisberg's TMs also considerably reduce the risk for relapse.

Though I have not suffered from sciatica in 16 years, I have gone to Dr. Weisberg for other ailments. I had an injury to my ankle that I sustained when I was a child. At the time, an orthopedic surgeon treated the torn ligaments in my ankle by casting it for over a month. The prolonged stasis caused permanent arthritic changes, which I assumed would always cause me pain. Once again, Dr. Weisberg showed me TMs that eliminated the pain and improved mobility at the ankle.

Dr. Weisberg is truly unique in the field of chronic pain. Before our chance encounter, I believed—even with my years of medical training—that chronic pain would forever be a part of my life. Instead, I now have a means whereby I can successfully, if not permanently, relieve pain when or if it should arise. His TMs should always be used to reduce the symptoms caused by daily wear and tear, heal microtraumatic and macrotraumatic injuries, and even, when appropriate, help ensure a successful recovery after surgical procedures. If done as directed, everyone (except those with disease or catastrophic trauma) can live a pain-free life.

8: The 3-Month Tune-Up: Monitor Your Machine

Who it's for: **Everyone**

Goal: **To tune up and monitor musculoskeletal health from head to toe**

Bonus Benefits: **Prevents minor problems from becoming acute or chronic pain**

THE HUMAN BODY IS A LIVING MACHINE. Like all other mechanical devices, its ability to function is determined by the specific condition of the individual parts that compose it. And like all other mechanical devices, the components that compose it can become worn, damaged, and defective with use. To counteract the destructive effects of wear and tear, the parts need to be regularly examined, tested, and repaired. It's probably safe to say that you regularly monitor and evaluate the condition of your car, but do you do the same for your body? While I'm sure you go to the doctor for regular *checkups* to evaluate your health, when was the last time you took your body in for a *tune-up* to evaluate your musculoskeletal health? Have you ever?

All mechanical devices need tune-ups from time to time to extend their lifetime durability. That's because no matter how well you take care of them, little things happen that can impair their performance. For instance, your car hits bumps in the road, dips into potholes, and carries the burden of excess loads. Its fan belt loosens, its oil becomes soiled, and its shock absorbers and brake pads wear down and erode. Your car may look and run fine, but on a deeper, mechanical level, these minor defects, if ignored, will eventually threaten the life of your vehicle.

The same holds true for the human body. It too hits bumps in the road, twists its ankles in potholes, and carries the burden of excess loads, such as body weight and objects. Its musculature shortens or elongates, its joints are underlubricated, and its disc shock absorbers and cartilage padding wear down and erode. You may look fit and feel that you are in perfect health, but on a deeper, biomechanical level, these minor injuries and dysfunctions, if ignored, will eventually cause your body to break down and fall into a painful state of disrepair. How can you prevent the debilitating accumulation of problems so small that they produce few or no symptoms and fail to register on your sensory radar screen? The answer is simple: You *test* for them.

The human body is its own mechanic. If you take it in for a tune-up, it will repair and heal itself.

The 3-Month Tune-Up adds greatly to the functional life of the human machine because it ascertains the functional condition of your musculoskeletal system, determines what adjustments need to be made, and immediately fixes any hidden problems it uncovers. It is an inventory in which you run through a checklist of body parts and perform a series of specially formulated diagnostic tests to see if everything is in good working order. Each diagnostic test includes explanations of what you are testing for, detailed instructions on how to proceed, and a pass/fail analysis. These tests are designed to challenge your muscles and joints to produce their intended movement without limitation, pain, or strain. If you meet the challenge, this establishes that the targeted muscles are at their optimal length and the targeted joints are expressing their full range of motion. If you pass, you will be directed to move on to the next body part. Alternately, if you do not meet the challenge, this establishes the presence of an underlying dysfunction or injury in the region that needs to be addressed. If you fail, you will be directed to amend the diagnostic test, turning it into corrective treatment and immediately initiating healing. You will re-peat these corrective treatments in conjunction with the 3-Minute Maintenance Method daily until you get a clean bill of health.

Many people have asked me why it is necessary to tune up their muscu-loskeletal system when they have already incorporated my maintenance program into their daily routine. This is a very good question. Here's why:

The 3-Minute Maintenance Method brings about optimal musculoskeletal health by targeting all of the major joints and muscle groups that require daily maintenance. But what of the anatomical areas that do not require regular and rig-orous maintenance yet are nonetheless susceptible to dysfunction and injury, such as the jaw? You need to test and service these remaining areas from time to time as well. Thus the 3-Month Tune-Up is the perfect complement for my daily pro-gram because it stops the progression of silently destructive minor injuries, and by catching them early, ensures that their repair is made with little time and effort. Once all of your body parts pass, you can return to maintaining the optimal con-dition of your musculoskeletal system in just three minutes a day.

You are almost ready to begin. But before you proceed there are a few im-portant do's and don'ts that I need to establish.

Do the Tune-Up Every Three Months

Most minor musculoskeletal dysfunctions and injuries produce few or no symp-toms and may therefore be easily ignored. While some of these will heal on their own and leave no residual by-products, others will not. In my experience as a prac-titioner, I have consistently observed that it takes approximately three months for the ramifications of minor dysfunctions and injuries to become apparent. Because of that, it would be uninformative to test the musculoskeletal system weekly or even monthly. On the other hand, I have found that a period longer than three months gives the injuries too much time to develop. Because musculoskeletal dysfunction always worsens with time, initially inconsequential injuries will steadily progress to more serious ailments. The longer a dysfunction is allowed to progress, the more intervention is needed to repair it. Thus monitoring your system every three months with a tune-up is the most practical way to catch minor musculoskeletal dysfunctions and injuries before it's too late.

Do Record and Save the Results of Your Tune-Ups

I have provided you with an inventory checklist on page 289 (Appendix) to help keep track of the results of your diagnostic tests. This is an important part of the tune-up process because it ensures that you will remember which body parts need to be temporarily included in your daily routine. The checklist also helps you to keep track of the date of your last tune-up and when your body is due for the next one. Finally, a written record allows you to do a careful analysis of previous tests. This can reveal important information about your musculoskeletal system. For instance, failure to pass a test once is an indication of a minor irritation that can be easily corrected; repeated failure indicates a more significant problem, usually an inherent defect in the area generally caused by one of the following or a combination thereof: an old injury whose residual scars prevent the region from returning to normal; an anatomical weak spot that is innately more vulnerable and susceptible to dysfunction; or overuse due to lifestyle or profession. Even if a defective area does not produce symptoms, it still needs the kind of substantial intervention provided for in the Encyclopedia of Pain Relief (see Chapter 7). By making note of repeated failure and targeting those body parts with specific therapeutic movements, you increase the likelihood of avoiding the crippling effects of dysfunctions and injuries in the future.

Do *Not* Take Your Body in for a Tune-Up before You've Engaged in the Daily Maintenance Program for Three Months

Whether you're a couch potato, weekend sportsperson, or top athlete, you've probably neglected to establish musculoskeletal health from a *biomechanical* point of view. But that's exactly the state your body needs to be in before attempting the tune-up. Why? The 3-Month Tune-Up is designed to make small modifications and adjustments to a healthy and functional musculoskeletal system. Until you have reached that level, you will probably fail most of the following diagnostic tests. Instead of being useful and instructive, the results will leave you frustrated and overwhelmed. While administering the tests cannot hurt, it will be more helpful to optimize the condition of your musculoskeletal system by actively engaging in the 3-Minute Maintenance Method for a period of three months before getting the tune-up for the first time.

Do *Not* Administer a Diagnostic Test on a Body Part That Already Has Symptoms

The purpose of the following diagnostic tests is to uncover imperceptible dysfunctions and injuries. If a body part already exhibits symptoms, there is nothing to test for. The problem is already clearly revealing itself through pain, inflammation, or limited mobility. Dysfunctions and injuries that have progressed to this stage are best dealt with by using the Encyclopedia of Pain Relief (Chapter 7). The corrective treatments in this chapter can be done in conjunction with the therapeutic movements in the Encyclopedia of Pain Relief. In fact, doing them together will help healing and ensure the most rapid relief. If you elect to do double duty, skip the diagnostic portion of the symptomatic body part and proceed directly to its corrective treatment. Then proceed with the remaining asymptomatic body parts until the tune-up is complete.

The 3-Month Tune-Up

Jaw

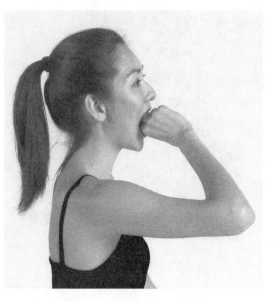

8–1. Jaw: Test and Treatment

DIAGNOSTIC TEST: To be able to open and close the jaw is necessary for survival because it permits two of the most basic human functions: consumption and communication. To eat and speak, the jaw needs to produce movement effortlessly and free of pain or restriction. When optimally functional, the jaw is able to open to the approximate width of two knuckles. To check this, insert the bent knuckles of your index and middle fingers in your mouth (see 8–1). Keep your jaw open wide enough so that your teeth are not pressed into the flesh of your fingers. Hold for five seconds. If you can do this free of strain or pain, you do not have an underlying dysfunction in the jaw and you pass. Move to the next body part.

CORRECTIVE TREATMENT: If opening your mouth to the width of two knuckles causes you to feel pain, you have uncovered an underlying dysfunction in the jaw joint. If it causes you to feel strain, the muscle of mastication (chewing muscle) is not at its optimal muscle length (O.M.L.). Failure to pass this test may also be an indication that you have TMJ, a common, often reversible musculoskeletal disorder of the jaw (see pages 157–158 for more information).

To correct the dysfunction, amend the diagnostic test by placing only the bent knuckle of your index finger in your mouth. Hold for 30 seconds. With each successive attempt, try to increase the opening of your jaw, going up to the point of pain but not past it. Repeat daily until you pass.

Neck

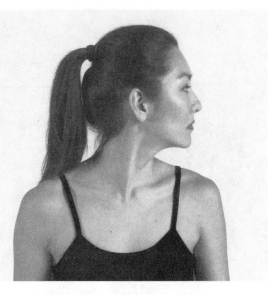

8–2. Neck: Test and Treatment

DIAGNOSTIC TEST: The neck is designed to permit movement of the head in a variety of ways: backward and forward, side to side, and turning (rotation). The most revealing way to assess the muscles and joints of the neck is by challenging its ability to fully rotate since nearly all movement in the neck involves rotation. When the neck is optimally functional, it is able to rotate 80 degrees to both left and right. To check this, turn your head to the left so that it is in alignment with your left shoulder (see 8–2). You will know that your neck has rotated 80 degrees when you are able to see behind you out of the corner of your eye. It is imperative that you keep your upper body—especially your shoulders—motionless. Hold for five seconds. Do the same turning to the right. If you can do this free of strain or pain, you pass. Move to the next body part.

CORRECTIVE TREATMENT: If you cannot turn your head a full 80 degrees or if doing so causes you strain or pain, you have uncovered an underlying dysfunction in the neck. More specifically, pain is usually an indication that the facet joints of the neck are improperly aligned, insufficiently lubricated, or damaged. Strain is an indication that the muscles of the region are not at their O.M.L.

To correct the dysfunction, amend the diagnostic test by turning your head as far as you can in the direction that produced the symptoms to the point of pain but not past it. Hold for 30 seconds. With each successive attempt, try to increase the rotation. Repeat daily until you pass.

Shoulders

DIAGNOSTIC TEST: The shoulder is the most mobile joint in the body. This makes it highly susceptible to dysfunction since the more mobile a joint is, the more likely it is to be injured. The shoulder permits large movement in six distinct ways: up and down, side to side, and external and internal rotation. When optimally functional, the shoulder is able to rotate 90 degrees both externally and internally. To check this, stand with your back against a wall. Lift your arms to shoulder height, keeping them horizontal. With palms facing downward, bend your elbows and bring them back so that they touch the wall. From this starting position bring your forearms up 90 degrees so that the backs of your hands touch the wall (see 8–3a). Hold for five seconds. Next, bring your forearms down 180 de-

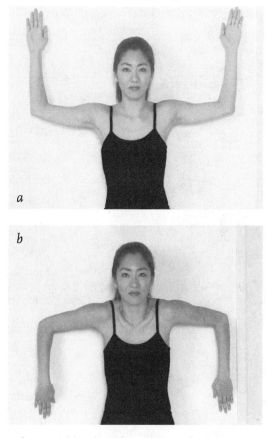

a

b

8–3a and b. Shoulders: Tests and Treatments

grees so that the palms of your hands touch the wall (see 8–3b). Make sure your shoulder blades maintain contact with the wall throughout the motion. Hold for five seconds. If you can do both motions without feeling strain or pain and without hearing body noises, such as popping, you pass. Move to the next body part.

CORRECTIVE TREATMENT: If either the upward or downward motion causes you to feel strain or pain or to hear body noises, one or both of your shoulder joints have limited mobility, your rotator cuff muscles are not at their O.M.L., or both.

To correct the dysfunction, amend the diagnostic test by moving your arms upward or downward to the maximum extent you can. Push up to the point of pain but not past it. Hold each position for 30 seconds. With each successive attempt, try to push your arms a little farther back against the wall. Repeat daily until you pass.

Elbows

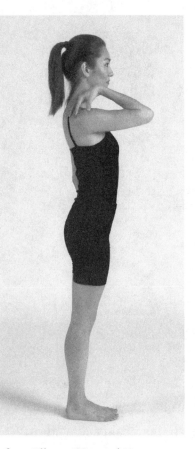

8–4. Elbows: Test and Treatment

DIAGNOSTIC TEST: The elbow is a very stable joint that is not prone to dysfunction, but the muscles that serve it are. Dysfunction in these muscles limits the full range of motion at the joint. When optimally functional, the muscles, specifically the triceps muscles, permit the bending of the elbow in toward the body to 145 degrees. To check this, extend your right arm straight out with your palm facing toward the ceiling. Bend your right arm so that your hand can grab the top of your right shoulder (see 8–4). Hold for five seconds. Repeat with the left arm. If you can do this motion without strain or pain, you pass. Move to the next body part.

CORRECTIVE TREATMENT: If you cannot bend your elbows enough to grab hold of your shoulders or if this causes you to feel strain or pain around the elbow, your triceps muscle is not at its O.M.L.

To correct the dysfunction, amend the diagnostic test by reaching back toward your shoulder as far as you can, to the point of pain but not past it. Hold for 30 seconds. With each successive attempt, try to increase the bending of the elbows. Repeat daily until you pass.

Wrists

DIAGNOSTIC TEST: The wrist, like the elbow, is served by the forearm muscles, which are highly prone to dysfunction. Moreover, unlike the elbow, the wrist itself is prone to dysfunction and injury because although it functions as a single joint, it is actually a conglomeration of eight carpal bones. (Most other joints in the body are made up of only two.) If the forearm muscle is not well maintained, it affects all eight of the bones in the wrist joint. When optimally functional, the short forearm muscles permit close to 90-degree angulation of the wrist. To check this, put your two palms together in a praying position (see 8–5). Raise your elbows so that your hands are perpendicular to the arms. Hold for five seconds. If you are able to assume this position without feeling strain or pain you pass. Move to the next body part.

CORRECTIVE TREATMENT: If you cannot assume a prayer position with your elbows raised, your short forearm muscles are not at their O.M.L. A limited range of motion in your wrists may also be indicative of the first stages of arthritis, synovitis, or a slight sprain. While failure to pass the test is not necessarily an indication of carpal tunnel syndrome, it may be an early warning sign that demands immediate attention (for more on this common musculoskeletal disorder, see page 167).

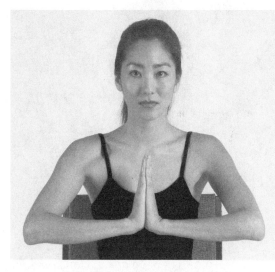

8–5. Wrists: Test and Treatment

To correct the dysfunction, amend the diagnostic test by raising your elbows as far as they can go to the point of pain but not past it. Hold for 30 seconds. With each successive attempt, try to increase the extent to which you raise your elbows. Repeat daily until you pass.

Hands and Fingers

DIAGNOSTIC TEST: The hands and fingers are able to accomplish the most intricate human endeavors, yet their major movements are limited to opening and closing. When the hands and fingers are optimally functional, they are able to open fully into a slight arch and close fully into a complete fist. To check this, open your hands, keeping your fingers straight and wide apart. Arch your hands backward so that there is a slight curve at the middle knuckle on all ten fingers (see 8–6a). Hold for five seconds. Next, make fists. Lay each thumb over and across the other four digits with the tip touching the ring finger (see 8–6b). Hold for five seconds. If you can arch your hands backward with no popping noises and can make fists free of pain, you pass. Move to the next body part.

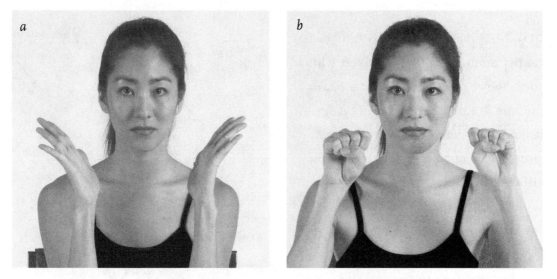

8–6a and b. Hands and Fingers: Tests and Treatment

CORRECTIVE TREATMENT: If you cannot arch your hands backward or make fists without pain, then the joints, the muscles in the region, or both are in dysfunction. This may also be an indication of the early stages of arthritic knuckles.

　　To correct the dysfunction, amend the first diagnostic test by opening your hands as far as you can up to the point of pain but not past it. Hold for 30 seconds. With each successive attempt, try to increase the degree of the arch. Next, amend the second portion of the diagnostic test by making fists, closing them as far as you can without pain. Squeeze and hold for 30 seconds. With each successive attempt, try to increase the closing of the fists. Repeat daily until you pass.

Upper Back

DIAGNOSTIC TEST: The upper back, specifically the thoracic spine, is less prone to dysfunction than many other areas in the body. However, the upper back as a whole, which contains 48 synovial joints, can suffer severe mechanical problems from acquired postural deviations. When the region is optimally functional, the muscles and joints of your shoulders and chest are flexible enough to permit optimal posture and to maintain it without rounded shoulders. To check this, stand with your feet shoulder-width apart. Place your toes inside the line of a doorway and put the palms of your hands on the door frame so that your upper arms are parallel to the floor. Lean forward until you feel your shoulder blades touch each other (see 8–7). Keep your head in alignment with your back; do not let your head tilt up or down, or lean forward or backward. Hold for five seconds. If you can do this motion without feeling any pain or strain, then you pass. Move to the next body part.

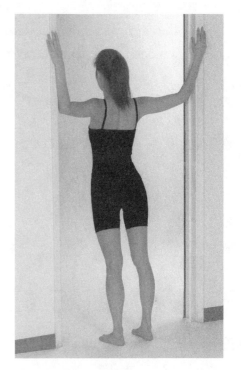

8–7. Upper Back: Test and Treatment

CORRECTIVE TREATMENT: If you cannot get your shoulder blades to touch, or if doing so produces strain or pain, the muscles of the upper back are in dysfunction. Failure to pass this test is an indication that the anterior musculature responsible for your posture is too tight and is thus contributing to acquired postural deviations in the spine.

To correct the dysfunction, amend the diagnostic test by leaning into the doorway as far as you can up to the point of pain but not past it. Hold for 30 seconds. With each successive attempt, try to lean in a little farther. Repeat daily until you pass.

Lower Back

DIAGNOSTIC TEST: Unlike the upper back, the lower back is one of the regions in the body most vulnerable to dysfunctions and injuries. This is because the burden of movement, under the weight of the body above it and anything else it carries, falls mostly here. The lower back permits mobility in many directions; they include bending forward, backward, and side to side. The best way to uncover a hidden dysfunction is to challenge its ability to rotate, because rotation plays an intimate role in the other possible movements of the region. When the lower back is optimally functional, it permits the rotating motion of turning the upper part of the body over the lower part. To check this, sit in a straight-backed chair with arm rests. Cross your left arm over your body and grab the right armrest (see 8–8). Pull as hard as you can so that your upper body is fully turned. You have reached the goal position when you are able to see behind you out of the corner of your eye. Be sure to keep your pelvis facing forward and your buttocks firmly fixed on the seat throughout. Hold for five seconds. Do the same motion turning to the left. If you can do this free of strain or pain, you pass. Move to the next body part.

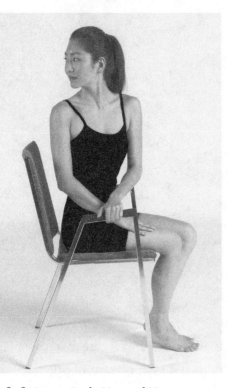

8–8. Lower Back: Test and Treatment

CORRECTIVE TREATMENT: If you cannot rotate far enough to see behind you or if doing so produces strain or pain, the muscles, joints, or both of the lower back are in dysfunction. Specifically, the musculature is not at its O.M.L., the joints are showing the early signs of arthritic changes, or both. Failure to pass this test may also be an indication of the first stages of a herniated disc (for more on this debilitating condition, see page 173).

To correct the dysfunction, amend the diagnostic test by turning as far as you can up to the point of pain but not past it. Hold for 30 seconds. With each successive attempt, try to pull a little harder, thus increasing the degree of rotation. Repeat daily until you pass.

Hips

DIAGNOSTIC TEST: The hip is second only to the shoulder in the amount of movement it permits. This makes it highly susceptible to biomechanical dysfunction, as is evident by the exceedingly high number of hip-replacement surgeries performed in the United States each year. The hip is the joint that connects the lower extremities to the rest of the body. When optimally functional, it permits the leg to rotate outwardly 45 degrees. To check this, sit in a straight-backed chair with your spine erect. Cross your right leg over your left knee at a 90-degree angle (see 8–9). Gently press on your right leg so that it is horizontal with the floor. To accurately assess the health of the joint, this motion must occur only at

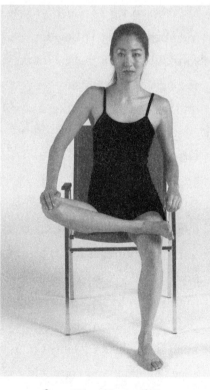

8–9. Hips: Test and Treatment

the hip. Therefore, keep your buttocks placed firmly on the seat and your hips in a fixed position; don't lift, tilt, or rotate your torso during the motion. Hold for five seconds. Repeat with the left leg crossed over the right knee. If you can get your leg into a horizontal position and it produces no strain or pain, you pass. Move to the next body part.

CORRECTIVE TREATMENT: If you cannot get your leg into a horizontal position without having to lift your buttocks off the chair or if it produces strain or pain, the function of your hip is compromised. Specifically, strain indicates short, tight muscles, and pain indicates inflammation or arthritic changes in the joints. Both conditions are very serious. If left untreated they will eventually erode the structure of the hips.

To correct the dysfunction, amend the diagnostic test by gently pressing on the crossed leg as much as you can up to the point of pain but not past it. Remember, no matter how far you can rotate the leg, it is imperative that you keep your buttocks on the seat of the chair for the duration of the motion. Hold for 30 seconds. With each successive attempt, try to push the crossed leg a little farther into the goal position. Repeat daily until you pass.

Knees

DIAGNOSTIC TEST: The knee is at a disadvantage, even under the best of conditions, because its construction favors mobility over stability. The large movements the knee permits, such as bending and straightening, are done without the protection of a fully restrictive encapsulation, so the musculature around the knee needs to be well maintained. Challenging the knee's active range of motion establishes the status of the musculature and the stability of the joint. When the knee is optimally functional, mobility occurs free of any muscle strain. To check this, sit on the edge of a chair and completely straighten your right leg so that your heel touches the floor (see 8–10a). Lift your left knee until your thigh touches your chest (see

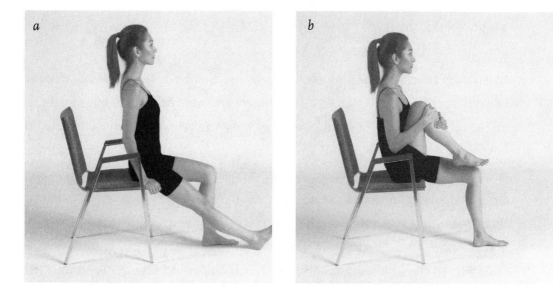

8–10a and b. Knees: Test and Treatment

8–10b). Use your arms to guide your leg inward and to press it as far into your chest as you can. Make sure your calf touches the back of your thigh. Hold for five seconds. Repeat with the left leg. If you can do this motion with ease, you pass. Move to the next body part.

CORRECTIVE TREATMENT: If you cannot bend your legs inward without strain or pain, the function in your knees is impaired. Specifically, the quadricep muscles are not at their O.M.L., the knee joints are unstable or arthritic, or both. Failure to pass this test may also be an indication that the meniscus (additional cartilage in the knees) is damaged.

To correct the dysfunction, amend the diagnostic test by bringing your legs in toward your body up to the point where it produce's strain or pain but not past it. Hold for 30 seconds. With each successive attempt, try to pull your leg a little closer to the goal position. Repeat daily until you pass.

Ankles

DIAGNOSTIC TREATMENT: The biggest threat to the ankles are small injuries. Little things that at the time seemed to be mere annoyances, such as missing a step off the curb or twisting your ankle while walking, can actually damage the tissue in the region. Although the painful symptoms of these small injuries quickly subside, residual scars remain. Unnoticed and left unresolved, these remnants cause mechanical dysfunction, making an already vulnerable area even more prone to injury. When optimally functional, the ankle permits an inward turning of 35 degrees, a motion that affords it the flexibility to withstand the most common jolting and awkward positions. To check this, stand with your feet shoulder-width apart. Bend your left ankle so that the outer portion of your left foot makes contact with the floor (see 8–11). Bear down on the ankle by putting weight on it. Hold for five seconds. Repeat with the right ankle. If doing this motion produces a feeling of strain—which it should—but not pain, you pass. Move to the next body part.

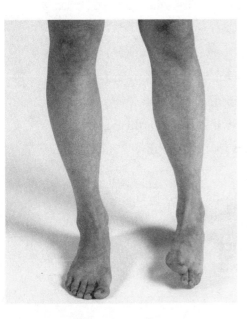

8–11. Ankles: Test and Treatment

CORRECTIVE TREATMENT: If bending your ankles inward causes pain, the length of the lateral muscles of the leg are not at their O.M.L. and the ankle joints are not able to move through their normal range of motion. Failure to pass this test is also an indication that residual scar tissue from previous injuries has accumulated in the tissues of the region.

To correct the dysfunction, amend the diagnostic test by bending your ankles to the extent that you feel strain but not pain. Hold for 30 seconds. With each successive attempt, try to push further toward the goal position. Repeat daily until you pass.

Feet and Toes

DIAGNOSTIC TEST: There are an infinite number of ways in which the muscles, bones, and joints that make up the feet and toes interact to create movement. The physics and mathematics that govern a single step are astonishing. When optimally functional, the feet and toes have the agility to instantaneously adapt to a vast spectrum of diverse terrain and do so free of pain. To check this, place a small hand towel flat on the floor. Stand on it and with a bare foot gather the towel together by pulling it toward your heels with your toes. Do this for five seconds or until the towel is in a little ball (see 8–12).

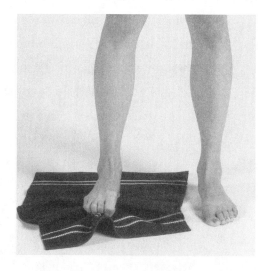

8–12. Feet and Toes: Test and Treatment

You should be able to gather approximately five inches in five seconds. Repeat with the opposite foot. If you can do this without producing a cramp, you pass.

CORRECTIVE TREATMENT: If you cannot gather a hand towel into a little ball without producing a cramp, your feet and toes do not have the ability to cope with their daily function.

To correct the dysfunction, amend the diagnostic test by slightly gathering the hand towel. Do this variation for 30 seconds or until you feel the onset of a cramp. With each successive attempt, try to gather the hand towel together a bit more than the previous try. Repeat daily until you pass.

Congratulations! You have now completed your tune-up. In doing so, you participated in the last of the three components of the Weisberg Way. As you can see, all aspects of my program work synergistically by approaching musculoskeletal health from every conceivable angle. If you continue to optimize your system with a daily application of the 3-Minute Maintenance Method, heal major injuries with the Encyclopedia of Pain Relief, and monitor and repair any minor dysfunction with the 3-Month Tune-Up, you will have gifted yourself with a fully pain-free life.

Happy Endings: Michelle's Story

Michelle R., age 40, is a perfect example of how people mistakenly equate the absence of musculoskeletal pain with the absence of musculoskeletal problems. Although she was healthy, physically fit, and pain free, she was in fact well on her way to a diminished quality of life.

I am one of the lucky few who never suffered any major bouts of musculoskeletal pain. While I've definitely had some minor aches and pains here and there throughout my life, none ever reached the level of debilitation that I've witnessed in so many of my family members, friends, co-workers, and acquaintances. Although I wasn't really sure why I was spared, I attributed it to the fact that I frequently take long hikes with my dogs, that my business keeps me on my feet and active, and that I eat pretty well. More than anything though, it seemed like a roll of the dice. And if I didn't know why I hadn't been in pain, I certainly didn't know how to prevent it from happening one day. In fact, the only thing I was sure of was that eventually my luck would run out. That's how I felt until I started doing the 3-Minute Maintenance Method and the 3-Month Tune-Up.

I became familiar with Dr. Weisberg's methods through his coauthor, Heidi Shink. She explained to me that if I wanted to remain pain free, I would have to maintain my musculoskeletal health and to do so in ways that exercise and lifestyle alone could not. She likened the Weisberg Way to a recipe, one of the main ingredients being the 3-Month Tune-Up (the other being the 3-Minute Maintenance Method). From the very start I loved doing the tune-up. Here was a way for me to check up on my body without having to go to a doctor or specialist. The tune-up wasn't only easy, simple, and fast, but it also produced some startling results. The first time out I failed *five* body parts, even though I didn't have any symptoms that would indicate that something was wrong. I was really shocked to discover that without even knowing it I had developed some musculoskeletal conditions that could eventually cause me enormous pain. I immediately began using the diagnostic tests as corrective treatments and did so until I passed. That was almost two years ago, and I haven't missed a tune-up yet.

I am happy to report that since I began the program I have remained pain free. Even more important, the little aches and pains that used to come and go without warning are no longer a part of my life. One of the most significant benefits of doing the tune-up regularly is knowing that I have control over determining the quality of my musculoskeletal health. I now have a way to help reveal problems that otherwise would have remained hidden until it was too late. The 3-Month Tune-Up is unique tool (I know of no other like it) that gives me a realistic assessment and deeper awareness of my body.

Part III

Special Circumstances

9: The Modified 3-Minute Maintenance Method

Who it's for: **Athletes, pregnant women, children (ages 5 to 15), and senior citizens**

Goal: **To provide optimal musculoskeletal health for people in special circumstances**

Bonus Benefits: **Prevents injuries, improves function, and increases performance for each group**

ALL HUMAN BEINGS PHYSIOLOGICALLY are primarily the same. Thus the design and function of our muscles and joints does not vary from person to person. What makes us unique are the ways that we emphasize or deemphasize different aspects of our bodies. While our musculoskeletal systems share common biological needs that must be met daily by maintaining optimal muscular length and taking joints through their full range of motion, our different physical circumstances can change the way in which we provide for those needs. I have identified four groups of people who, for reasons of lifestyle choices, activities, or age, must be challenged on their own level so that they too can live a pain-free life.

The 3-Minute Maintenance Method provides the foundation for optimal musculoskeletal health for most people. However, there are some whose physicality deviates so far from the norm that they cannot perform my general program in an appropriate and meaningful way. These people fall into four groups: athletes, pregnant women, children (ages 5 to 15), and senior citizens. High-performance athletes are usually too strong and flexible to benefit from my general program, and senior citizens are usually too weak and inflexible. Pregnant women have a temporarily reduced physical capacity, rendering parts of the program impossible, and children have a temporarily heightened physical capacity, rendering parts of the program insufficient. To achieve the same goals as I had for the general population, I accounted for the differences by making specific changes tailored for each group. The result is the Modified 3-Minute Maintenance Method, one for each of the four groups of people with special circumstances.

The Modified 3-Minute Maintenance Method consists of six different therapeutic movements (TMs) that target all major muscle groups and joints. Although most of the targeted areas are identical to my general program, the modifications enhance and emphasize different areas according to each group's needs. To understand why I've made the modifications and which areas most benefit from them, I have provided a list and an analysis of the individual changes. (For a complementary analysis of the original TMs, refer back to Chapter 6, starting on page 132.) I have also provided instructions on how to do each TM correctly and safely.

Before you begin your specialized program, you should remember that the following TMs represent goal positions. If you are unable to do one or more of the TMs fully at first or if doing so causes you pain, use your limitations as a guide and let your body dictate what your starting point should be. With consistent daily application, you will eventually work your way to the goal positions. Be patient with the pace at which you progress and you will reap the rewards of optimal musculoskeletal health.

The Modified 3-Minute Maintenance Method: Athletes

Athletes come in all shapes and sizes, and they engage in a wide variety of sports. The diverse spectrum of athleticism accounts for the different physical strengths and weaknesses that emphasize various components of the musculoskeletal system. Some athletes, such as tennis players, overdevelop their upper extremities, while some, such as runners, overdevelop their lower extremities. Still others, such as gymnasts, overdevelop both their upper and lower extremities. On the other hand, some athletes, such as ballet dancers, increase their flexibility, while some, such as weight lifters, reduce their flexibility. Still others, such as football players, both increase and reduce their flexibility at the same time.

Unique Goals and Bonus Benefits

- **Supertunes the athlete's musculoskeletal system**
- **Prevents common injuries associated with athletes**
- **Improves athletic performance**

In spite of the diversity, all athletes require a higher level of musculoskeletal performance because of the intensified demand placed on their systems. The consequence of this intensification is that all athletes have more of an imperative than the rest of us to maintain the optimal condition of their muscles and joints.

Unfortunately, athleticism is not synonymous with musculoskeletal health. Many athletes I've treated are so focused on perfecting their specializations that they failed to learn how to maintain the basics. That is why so many athletes are constantly plagued by *preventable* injuries. High force and impact, coupled with dysfunctional muscles and joints, make athletes more vulnerable to both macro-traumatic and microtraumatic injuries than the average person. The Modified 3-Minute Maintenance Method is designed to establish the foundation of musculoskeletal health for athletes by challenging them with a level of difficulty that corresponds to their needs.

1. Modified Bow for Athletes

TARGETED AREAS: Spine, elbows, hands, fingers, knees, hips, shins, and ankles

MODIFIED TARGETED AREAS: Rotator muscle groups of the shoulders and hips

INSTRUCTIONS: Kneel down on the floor and seat your buttocks on your heels. Your legs should be approximately hip-width apart. Rotate your feet outward so that your toes point away from your body. Bend over and reach forward as far as you can, keeping your arms and elbows straight and shoulder-width apart. Place your palms flat on the floor and rotate them outward so that the insides of your hands face away from your body (see 9–1). Your head should be slightly elevated in a comfortable and neutral position. Hold for 30 seconds.

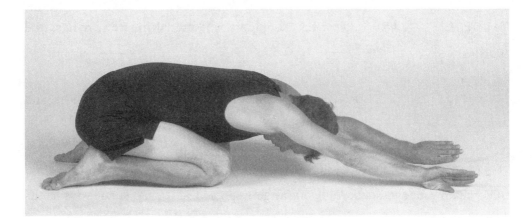

9–1. Modified Bow for Athletes

ANALYSIS: As an athlete, you subject your muscles and joints to greater forces, which means that they need to be challenged with greater precision and intensity. The Bow covers a lot of physiological ground. This TM provides the foundation for the stability of the entire body by focusing on the spine while enhancing the bio-mechanics and functional health of additional targeted areas (see previous page). The Modified Bow for Athletes increases the level of demand and difficulty by adding rotation to the upper and lower extremities. Because the muscles and joints that engage in these modified motions are intimately involved in almost all high-performance athletics, they are also among the most vulnerable to injury. By stretching the rotator cuff muscles of the shoulders and the rotator muscles of the hips, you restore their optimal muscle length (O.M.L.), which reduces their impo-sition on the respective joints. Stretching these muscles also stops the buildup of microtraumas in these regions, indirectly minimizes the likelihood of macro-traumatic injuries, such as sprains, strains, and dislocations, and heightens your athletic ability and performance.

2. Modified Arch for Athletes

TARGETED AREAS: Spine, neck, shoulders, abdominal muscles, hands, and fingers

MODIFIED TARGETED AREAS: Forearm muscles, elbows, wrists, knees, and ankles

INSTRUCTIONS: Kneel and lean forward, placing your palms flat on the floor underneath your shoulders with your fingers spread wide apart. Rotate your hands inward so that your fingers point toward each other and rotate your feet outward so that your toes point away from each other. Keep your back and head straight. Slowly arch your back upward (see 9–2a), while lowering your head. Then reverse the movement. Slowly arch your back downward (see 9–2b), while raising your head. This continuous motion should take three seconds. Do this 10 times for a total of 30 seconds.

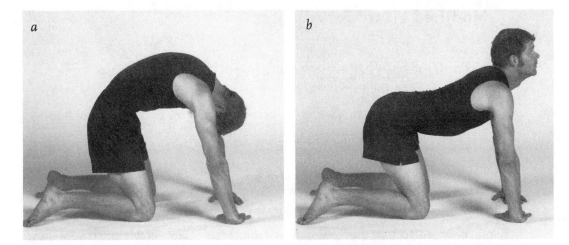

9–2a and b. Modified Arch for Athletes

ANALYSIS: The biological need to mobilize the spine is fundamental to all people; for the athlete, who uses his or her body more rigorously, it is absolutely essential. The Arch takes the spine through its full range of motion, lubricating and nourishing the spinal facet joints while enhancing the biomechanical and functional health of additional targeted areas (see previous page). The Modified Arch for Athletes increases the level of demand and difficulty by adding rotation to the upper and lower extremities. The emphasis is on the length of the forearm muscles and the agility of those that govern the movement of the knees and ankles. Most athletes place enormous demands on their forearm muscles. In order to prevent wear and tear, and injury to the elbows and wrists, the optimal length of these muscles must be well maintained. By rotating the hands inward, you stretch the forearm muscles, thereby restoring their O.M.L. Most athletes also need their knees and ankles to be very agile. By rotating the feet outward, you stretch the muscles that are intimately involved with the knees and ankles, restoring their O.M.L. and diminishing the impact of high-performance activities.

3. Modified Lizard for Athletes

TARGETED AREAS: Spine (specifically, the discs) and lower back

MODIFIED TARGETED AREAS: Rotator muscle groups of the shoulders and hips

INSTRUCTIONS: Lie on your stomach. Place your palms flat on the floor slightly wider than shoulder-width apart, spread your fingers wide, and rotate your hands outward so that they point away from each other. Slowly push your head and shoulders up until your elbows are straight and look up toward the ceiling. Your palms should end up underneath your shoulders. Rotate your feet inward so that your toes point toward each other (see 9–3). Hold for 30 seconds.

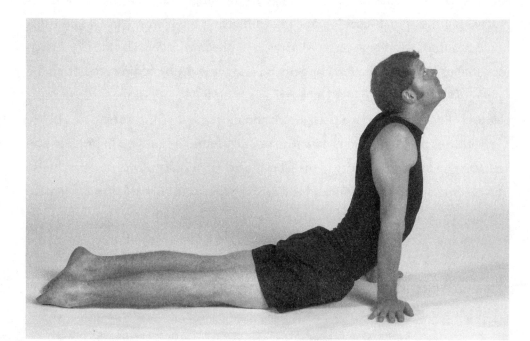

9–3. Modified Lizard for Athletes

ANALYSIS: Under normal lifestyle conditions, the discs that are sandwiched between the spinal vertebrae are highly vulnerable to a painful and debilitating condition known as a slipped disc. The disc's vulnerability to protrusion, bulging, and herniation is magnified exponentially by high-performance athleticism. The Lizard stretches the anterior paraspinal muscles around the discs most at risk, pushing them back to their optimal position. This reduces both the likelihood of injury and stress on the lower back. The Modified Lizard for Athletes raises the level of difficulty by rotating the upper and lower extremities in the opposite direction of the previous TMs. As an athlete, you cannot overemphasize rotation: Almost all athletes suffer injuries due to limitations in their rotator muscles. By changing the direction of the stretch, you cover all possible causes of dysfunction by fully restoring the O.M.L. of these vital muscle groups.

4. Modified Natural Squat for Athletes

TARGETED AREAS: Lower back, pelvis, knees, and ankles

MODIFIED TARGETED AREAS: Hips and postural control

INSTRUCTIONS: Place your feet two inches apart and squat. Keep your heels flat on the ground. Raise your arms above your head shoulder-width apart and straighten your back (see 9–4). Keep your head level so that your chin does not tilt downward or upward. Hold for 30 seconds.

ANALYSIS: Squatting is one of the most therapeutic ways to move your body. The Natural Squat takes the lower back, pelvis, hips, knees, and ankles through their full range of motion, thereby lubricating these vital joints, and stretches their corresponding musculature, thus restoring O.M.L. The Modified Natural Squat for Athletes considerably raises the bar on this TM. By placing your feet close together, you increase the challenge to the mobility of your hips. By raising your hands above your head, you increase the challenge to postural control.

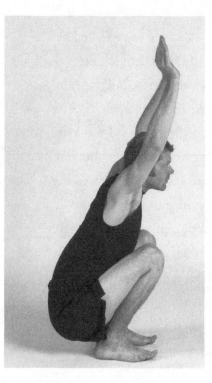

9–4. Modified Natural Squat for Athletes

An athlete's entire body is subject to high impact. To withstand the intensified demand free of injury and pain, your spine needs to be strengthened and balanced daily. The ability to do the Modified Natural Squat for Athletes is an indication of appropriate joint movement and muscle length, good physical coordination and biomechanics, and optimal postural control and body flexibility. Most athletes I've worked with over the years have trouble doing this TM fully at first because they have not established a foundation for musculoskeletal health. If you find that this TM is too difficult, modify it by spreading your legs a little farther apart and clasping your hands behind your head. Work up to the full position over time. After you reach the goal position, you should experience a dramatic reduction in injury, discomfort, and pain.

5. Modified Split for Athletes

TARGETED AREAS: Lower back, inner thigh muscles, and knees

MODIFIED TARGETED AREAS: Hips, pelvic girdle, and hamstring muscles

INSTRUCTIONS: Sit down on the floor, spread your legs as far apart as you can, and keep your knees straight (see 9–5a). Hold for 15 seconds. Next, bend forward at the lower back and touch your toes with your hands (see 9–5b). Hold for 15 seconds.

ANALYSIS: The modifications to this TM are the most radical of all. In my general program, the Split is primarily concerned with restoring the O.M.L. of the inner thigh muscles because the majority of the population suffers diminished flexibility

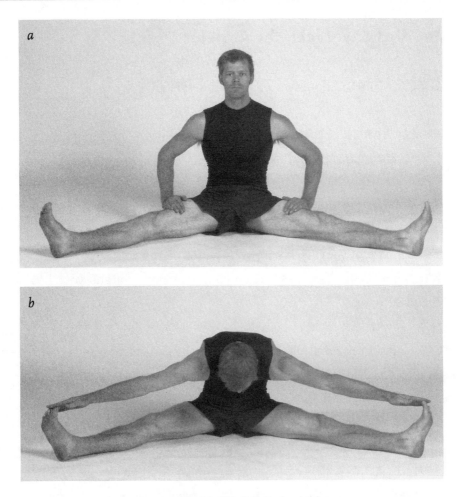

9–5a and b. Modified Split for Athletes

here. Most athletes' inner thigh muscles are so flexible that there is no need to challenge them this aggressively. By altering the position, the Modified Split for Athletes maintains the flexibility of this muscle group without overloading it. Moreover, the change of position also increases the challenge by increasing the number of targeted muscles. Bending forward stretches the hamstring muscles, which helps to protect the knees from injury during high-impact athletics. It also frees any muscular restrictions in the pelvic girdle, greatly adding to the functional life of the lower back. Finally, it stretches the muscles around the hips, reducing their imposition on these vital joints.

6. Modified Sky Reach for Athletes

TARGETED AREAS: Shoulders, elbows, and wrists

MODIFIED TARGETED AREAS: Spine (specifically, proper postural alignment), hips, knees, ankles, and feet

INSTRUCTIONS: Sit down on the floor, place the soles of your feet together, and press your knees downward. Raise your arms over your head, bend your elbows, and grab the base of your neck with your hands. Bring your elbows back so that your wing bones touch (see 9–6). Keep your spine straight and your head level. Hold for 30 seconds.

ANALYSIS: Proper postural alignment requires the participation and optimal health of a significant portion of the musculature from your lower back upward. The fundamental ability to maintain good posture through the Sky Reach is an indication that the paraspinal muscles are appropriately strong. The Modified Sky Reach for Athletes increases the postural challenge by having you grab the base of your neck. This position stretches the rotator cuffs, which are the single most vulnerable muscle group for athletes, thus restoring their O.M.L. It also takes the shoulder and elbow joints through a full range of motion and strengthens the wrist flexor muscles by maintaining the position. My general program focuses primarily on the upper extremities in the Sky Reach; the Modified Sky Reach for Athletes adds emphasis to the lower extremities. An athlete's hips are subjected to tremendous forces, so there is a greater mandate to provide

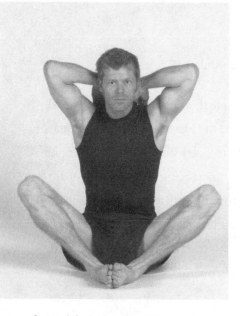

9–6. Modified Sky Reach for Athletes

for their biological needs. By placing the soles of your feet together and bringing your knees down toward the floor, you challenge the rotation of the hip joints. This enhances the hips' mobility, which is crucial for the optimal function of the knees. This position also stretches and strengthens the musculature in your legs and provides additional stability for the knees, ankles, and feet.

The Modified 3-Minute Maintenance Method: Pregnancy

The natural phenomenon of pregnancy is a temporary imposition on a woman's body. Like an athlete, a pregnant woman requires a higher level of musculoskeletal performance because of the intensified demand placed on her system. A healthy pregnancy changes a woman's body configurations for 12 months (9 months of pregnancy, 3 months of recovery), reduces what she can do physically, and increases musculoskeletal dysfunction. The increase in weight is carried mostly by her knees and feet, the fetal position affects her lower back, and the hormonal changes and general level of stress tighten and restrict the musculature throughout her body. All of this, coupled with a woman who goes into pregnancy without a high level of musculoskeletal health, makes for a difficult and often painful ordeal that can extend beyond the birth of her baby. Physical limitations, injuries, and pain during pregnancy induce physiological reactions, such as muscle spasms and cramps, that compromise the situation even more, make delivery harder, and leave recovery incomplete.

Unique Goals and Bonus Benefits

- **Maintains and enhances physical abilities while reducing the stress of pregnancy**
- **Prevents injuries associated with pregnancy**
- **Prepares the body for a natural and healthy delivery**

Pregnancy does not have to be catastrophic to a woman's body. Our female ancestors (and women who live similarly today) suffered almost no musculoskeletal ramifications of pregnancy because they moved more and did so appropriately.

The Modified 3-Minute Maintenance Method is designed to reduce the trauma of pregnancy and delivery by optimizing musculoskeletal health. While the biological needs of a pregnant woman are no different from what they were before she was expecting, the TMs emphasize areas that are rendered more vulnerable at this unique time. The TMs have also been altered to accommodate the enlargement of the womb, making the program safe for both mother and child.

1. Modified Bow for Pregnancy

TARGETED AREAS: Spine, shoulders, elbows, hands, fingers, hips, knees, shins, and ankles

MODIFIED TARGETED AREAS: Pelvis

INSTRUCTIONS: Kneel on the floor and seat your buttocks on your heels. Spread your knees approximately three feet apart or just beyond shoulder width. Bend over and reach forward as far as you can. Place your palms flat on the floor and spread your fingers wide apart, keeping your arms shoulder-width apart (see 9–7). Your

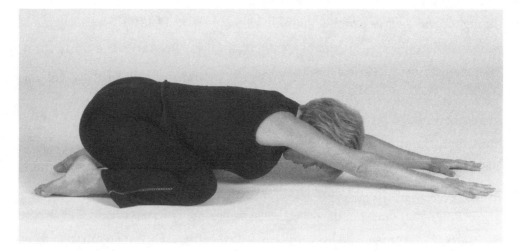

9–7. Modified Bow for Pregnancy

arms and elbows should be straight and your head should be slightly elevated in a comfortable and neutral position. Hold for 30 seconds.

ANALYSIS: Many women are encouraged to move less during pregnancy. The consequences of this poor advice are dysfunctional muscles and joints, which limit physical capabilities and increase the likelihood of injury and pain. You don't need to move less, you just need to prepare your muscles and joints for the increased imposition so that you can move both risk free and pain free. Establishing optimal musculoskeletal health always starts with the spine. For the pregnant woman whose increased fetal weight overburdens the spine, this is especially critical. The Bow releases and relieves the stress on the spine by taking its facet joints through their full range of motion and stretching the muscles that run its entire length. This TM also prepares your body for the increased imposition of pregnancy by targeting muscles and joints in both your upper and lower extremities (see previous page). The Modified Bow for Pregnancy has one significant change from my general program: the parting of your knees to accommodate the enlargement of the womb. This stretches the pelvis, which helps to prepare for a safer and easier delivery. In all other respects, the benefits are identical.

2. Modified Arch for Pregnancy

TARGETED AREAS: Spine, neck, shoulders, abdominal muscles, forearm muscles, wrists, elbows, hands, and fingers

MODIFIED TARGETED AREAS: Hips and pelvic girdle

INSTRUCTIONS: Kneel and spread your knees approximately three feet apart, or just beyond shoulder width. Turn your feet outward so that your toes point away from the body. Lean forward and place your palms flat on the floor underneath your shoulders, with your fingers spread wide apart. Keep your back and head straight. Slowly arch your back upward (see 9–8a) while lowering your head. Then

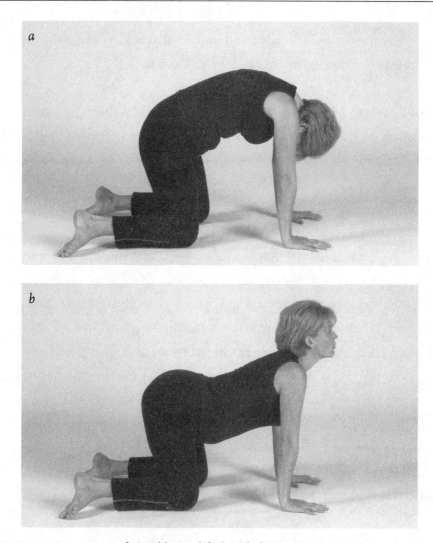

9–8a and b. Modified Arch for Pregnancy

reverse the movement. Slowly arch your back downward (see 9–8b) while raising your head. This continuous motion should take three seconds. Do this 10 times for a total of 30 seconds.

ANALYSIS: Once again we focus on the health of the spine, which is so important during pregnancy, with the emphasis here on mobilizing the spinal joints. The Arch takes these joints from one end of their range of motion to the other while stretching the paraspinal muscles that run along the length of the entire structure. The fluid motion also strengthens the abdominal muscles, further increasing the stability of the lower back. Finally, the Arch enhances the biomechanics and functional health of additional targeted areas (see page 231).

The Modified Arch for Pregnancy targets the unique concerns of pregnancy by spreading the knees to accommodate the enlarged womb and rotating the feet outward. The rotation of the lower extremities has two important benefits. First, it stretches the muscles around the hips, which are extremely vulnerable to the increased stress of pregnancy. The elongation reduces the buildup of microtraumas around these joints and reduces their susceptibility to dysfunction, injury, and pain. Second, the rotation stretches the entire pelvic region, increasing pelvic flexibility, to facilitate a healthier, easier, and safer delivery.

3. Modified Lizard for Pregnancy

TARGETED AREAS: Spine (specifically, the discs), lower back, neck, shoulders, forearms, thumbs, and ankles

MODIFIED TARGETED AREAS: Standing position to accommodate enlargement of the womb

INSTRUCTIONS: Stand with your feet shoulder-width apart. Grasp the top of your pelvis with your thumbs facing forward and your fingers spread across the small of your lower back. Gently push your lower back forward (see 9–9). Lift your chest toward the ceiling and let your head, shoulders, and legs follow the lead of the arch, stopping when you see the ceiling directly above you. Hold for 30 seconds.

ANALYSIS: The lower back, already one of the most vulnerable regions in the body, is the most common source of dysfunction, injury, and pain during pregnancy. That is because the increased up-front weight throws off the delicate mus-

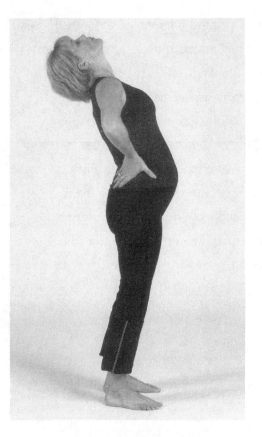

9–9. Modified Lizard for Pregnancy

culoskeletal balance in this area. Furthermore, to accommodate the changing bodily configurations over the nine-month period, the musculature in the lower back tightens up and shortens around the spine. This imposes upon the lumbar spinal vertebrae and overburdens the corresponding discs that lie between them, which can cause them to protrude, herniate, or even rupture. The Lizard eliminates these serious problems by stretching the muscles in the lower back in a horizontal position. The Modified Lizard for Pregnancy produces the same benefits in a standing position. This TM restores the O.M.L. of the muscles in your lower back while pushing the discs back to their optimal positions. The bonus in relieving pressure from the lower back is that it relieves pressure from the womb. The Modified Lizard for Pregnancy also stretches the muscles in your neck, shoulders, forearms, thumbs, and ankles, making their corresponding joints more stabilized.

4. Modified Natural Squat for Pregnancy

TARGETED AREAS: Lower back

MODIFIED TARGETED AREAS: Pelvis, hips, knees, and ankles

INSTRUCTIONS: Spread your legs just beyond shoulder-width apart, toes pointing slightly outward, and squat (see 9–10). Keep your heels flat on the floor. You may have your arms in any position—resting on your knees as shown or straight out in front of you—but do not use any external devices for balance. Hold for 30 seconds.

ANALYSIS: Most of the pregnant women I've treated over the years think that squatting is not only impossible to do in their condition but also harmful. In fact, the opposite is true. A pregnant woman should be able to squat effortlessly, and doing so is beneficial for both the duration of the pregnancy and delivery. For thousands of years our ancestors assumed a squatting position to give birth, and many health care professionals still recommend this practice.

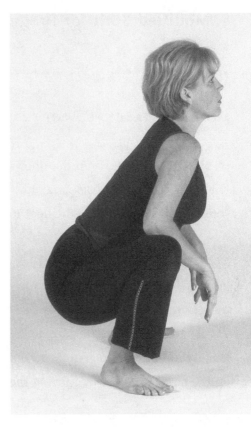

9–10. Modified Natural Squat for Pregnancy

The Natural Squat offsets the deficiency of lifestyle by supplementing the biological needs of your lower back, pelvis, hips, knees, and ankles. The Modified Natural Squat for Pregnancy enhances the external rotation of the lower extremities by having you spread your knees farther apart than in my general program. This allows for the growing womb and reduces stress in the lower regions of your body, which helps to prevent the swelling in the ankles and feet that commonly occurs during pregnancy. This modification also stretches the pelvis more completely, thereby enhancing the flexibility and performance of the muscles and joints in this region during delivery.

5. Modified Split for Pregnancy

TARGETED AREAS: Hips and knees

MODIFIED TARGETED AREAS: Inner thigh muscles and groin region

INSTRUCTIONS: Sit on the floor and spread your legs as far apart as you can. Keep your knees and back straight and point your toes upward (see 9–11). Place your hands behind you on the floor for additional support. Hold for 30 seconds.

ANALYSIS: Next to the lower back, the hips and knees are most at risk during pregnancy. In my general program, the Split targets the knees by stretching the musculature most intimately involved with supporting and protecting them. This TM then targets the hip region by mobilizing it in a bent position. The addition of fetal weight during pregnancy makes both of these positions too much of a strain on the targeted areas. By moving the position to the floor, the Modified Split for

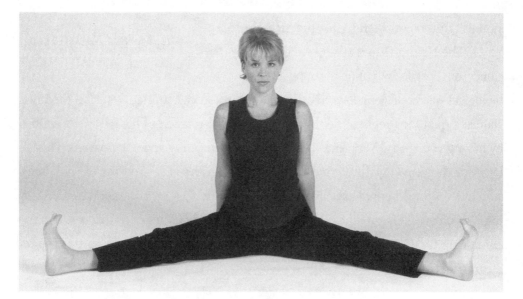

9–11. Modified Split for Pregnancy

Pregnancy stretches the inner thigh and groin muscle groups without overloading them yet still benefits the hips and knees. The change of position also facilitates the health of the hips by simulating the bend of the trunk through sitting. Finally, by pointing your toes upward, you stretch the Achilles tendon, which benefits the ankles. The modifications represent a safe way to provide for the same biological needs met by the Split.

6. Modified Sky Reach for Pregnancy

TARGETED AREAS: Elbows, hips, knees, ankles, feet, and toes

MODIFIED TARGETED AREAS: Spine (specifically, proper postural alignment) and shoulders

INSTRUCTIONS: Assume a comfortable seated position on the floor with your legs crossed and curl your toes. Raise your arms up to shoulder height (see 9–12a), bend your elbows 90 degrees, and lift your hands so that your fingers point to the sky (see 9–12b). Hold for 30 seconds.

ANALYSIS: Maintaining proper postural alignment, which is fundamental to body mechanics and health, can be difficult during pregnancy. The additional weight in the lower regions of the body pulls on the spine, causing it to curve unnaturally. The consequences of this unnatural curvature are dysfunction, susceptibility to injury, and pain. The Sky Reach restores optimal posture through elongation and straightening of the spine. While the level of difficulty of the Modified Sky Reach for Pregnancy is slightly reduced from my general program—reaching the hands over the head would tug on the womb—it still effectively challenges the strength of the paraspinal muscles by having them hold up the weight of your arms for 30 seconds. The Modified Sky Reach for Pregnancy also lengthens and strengthens the rotator cuff muscles of the shoulders and the tri-

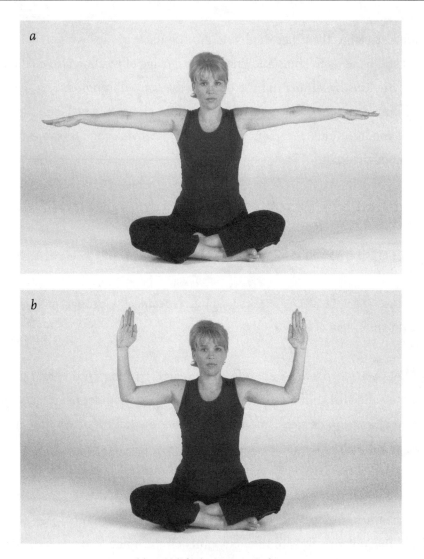

9–12a and b. Modified Sky Reach for Pregnancy

ceps muscles of the elbows, whose health will come in handy once your child is born—think of constantly picking the baby up and putting him or her down. Finally, this TM targets the lower extremities by stretching the rotator muscles of the hips, quadriceps muscles of the knees, dorsiflexor muscles of the ankles, and toe extensor muscles of the toes.

The Modified 3-Minute Maintenance Method: Children (Ages 5 to 15)

Childhood, like pregnancy, is a temporary condition. But unlike pregnancy, childhood is a heightened, rather than reduced, level of physicality. From birth to approximately five years of age, the human musculoskeletal system is highly fit and functional in large part because its biological needs are well served daily. The very young are extremely active, fully and appropriately utilize all their muscles and joints, and have a natural inclination to climb and squat. At five years of age, however, the cycle of musculoskeletal dysfunction, damage, and deterioration is set in motion because that is when children are indoctrinated into our sitting culture. They are encouraged to be seated for excessively long periods while at school, in class, at home for meals and homework, and even for leisure during video games and computer use. They move less, play less, and almost never climb or squat. Although children ages 5 to 15 still enjoy an increased level of agility, flexibility, and endurance, the natural benefits of youth are negated by the deficiencies of a modern lifestyle. The consequences of this are far worse than you may realize. Chronic and recurrent pain, once suffered mainly by those over 40, now affect some 10 million American children under the age of 18.[1] Arthritis, once labeled an old person's illness, is now known to begin its destructive path in the teens. And musculoskeletal injuries, such as sprains and strains, once seen only rarely in children, are increasingly prevalent.

Fortunately, children's muscles and joints are far more forgiving than those of adults and the deficiencies of their lifestyle can be effectively counteracted. The Modified 3-Minute Maintenance Method is designed to maintain children's heightened physical capabilities until their maturation process is complete. The TMs challenge children at their own unique level so that the biological needs of

---

Unique Goals and Bonus Benefits

■ **Maintains children's heightened physical condition**

■ **Diminishes the aches and pains of growing**

■ **Carries children into adulthood at a higher level of functioning**

their muscles and joints are provided daily. The program also preserves children's musculoskeletal health *before* problems set in. By nurturing and optimizing their systems in this way, while setting a good example by doing the 3-Minute Maintenance Method along with them, you turn their temporarily hightened musculoskeletal condition into a more lasting and permanent one that extends not only into their adulthood but also their senior years.

1. Modified Bow for Children

TARGETED AREAS: Spine, elbows, hands, fingers, hips, knees, shins, and ankles

MODIFIED TARGETED AREAS: Shoulders

INSTRUCTIONS: Kneel and seat your buttocks on your heels. Your inner thighs should be touching. Bend over and reach forward as far as you can, keeping your arms and elbows straight and shoulder-width apart. Place your forehead and palms on the floor. Spread your fingers wide apart and lift your arms off the floor so that they are the same height as the top of your head (see 9–13). Hold for 30 seconds.

ANALYSIS: Poor musculoskeletal health begins with poor musculoskeletal habits established in childhood. Although children don't usually suffer the consequences

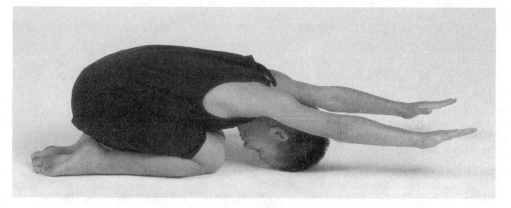

9–13. Modified Bow for Children

until they're older, sitting, immobility, and lack of proper musculoskeletal maintenance will play a significant role in their quality of life. But childhood presents an opportunity to stop problems before they start. This is particularly true when it comes to the spine. By establishing its health early in life, the plethora of corrections that must be made in adulthood—postural changes, vertebrae and disc realignment, and muscular rebalancing—can be effectively circumvented.

The Bow optimizes the health of the spine by mobilizing the spinal joints and stretching the paraspinal muscles (the five layers of muscle that run along its length and account for the vast majority of back pain in adults). Because a child's spine is more agile and flexible than an adult's, the demand must be increased to bring about the same biomechanical results. The Modified Bow for Children substantially increases the challenge. With the child's head on the floor, the curvature of the spine is extended and its health improved. By the child's raising his or her arms off the ground, the shoulder muscles are strengthened and the shoulder joints are stabilized. The benefits to the upper extremities (including elbows, hands, and fingers) and lower extremities (including the hips, knees, shins, and ankles) are identical to my general program.

2. Modified Arch for Children

TARGETED AREAS: Spine, neck, abdominal muscles, and hips

MODIFIED TARGETED AREAS: Shoulders, elbows, wrists, hands, fingers, and feet

INSTRUCTIONS: Come to a kneeling position and place the pads of your toes on the floor. Make fists and lean forward, placing the top of your fists on the floor underneath your shoulders. Keep your back and head straight. Slowly arch your back upward (see 9–14a) while lowering your head. Then reverse the movement. Slowly arch your back downward (see 9–14b) while raising your head. This continuous motion should take three seconds. Do this 10 times for a total of 30 seconds.

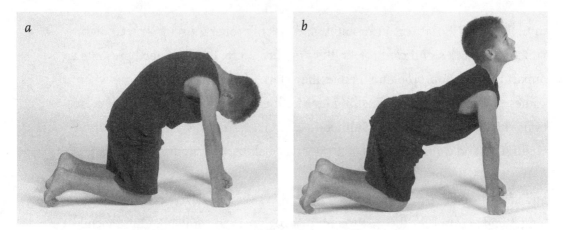

9–14a and b. Modified Arch for Children

ANALYSIS: The health of the spine is so important to lifelong body mechanics and function that we target it again with this TM. The Arch takes the spine, including the neck, through its full range of motion, ensuring that the facet joints are fully lubricated with nourishing synovial fluid. This TM also stretches the paraspinal muscles, restoring their O.M.L., while strengthening the abdominal muscles that contract and relax through the duration of the motion. Finally, it activates the muscles that stabilize the hip and shoulder joints.

The Modified Arch for Children increases the challenge by increasing the demands to children's upper and lower extremities. By placing the impact of body weight on the fists, as opposed to the flat hands in the general program, the child's shoulder and forearm muscles are strengthened, and hands, fingers, wrists, and elbows are stabilized. This is very important because our modern lifestyle no longer provides for the biological needs of the upper extremities. This TM anticipates adult problems and helps to thwart them by supplementing the limitations before their ramifications become permanent. By placing the weight of the lower body on the toes as opposed to flat legs in the general program, the child's feet are stretched. This is also very important as it counteracts the debilitating, cumulative effects of wearing shoes.

3. Modified Lizard for Children

TARGETED AREAS: Spine (specifically, the discs), neck, shoulders, elbows, wrists, hands, lower back, ankles, and feet

MODIFIED TARGETED AREAS: Quadriceps muscles and pelvic region

INSTRUCTIONS: Lie on your stomach. Place your palms flat on the floor and spread your fingers wide apart. Slowly push your head and shoulders up until your elbows are straight and look toward the ceiling. Your palms should end up underneath your shoulders. Bend your knees and bring your feet toward your head (see 9–15). Keep your lower stomach touching the floor throughout. Hold for 30 seconds.

ANALYSIS: The chronic aches and pains that plague the lower backs of most adults are usually the result of years of neglect. One of the most debilitating conditions occurs when irregularities in the spine push the discs sandwiched between the vertebrae to extend beyond their normal boundaries. While a child rarely suffers from a slipped disc, the seeds of dysfunction that cause its occurrence in later years are often sown early in life. The Lizard targets the spinal discs by stretching the musculature in the lower back. By pushing the discs back into normal position and maintaining their optimal placement during childhood, the likelihood of developing problems with them in adulthood is greatly reduced. The Lizard also enhances the overall biomechanics and functional health of additional targeted areas (see above).

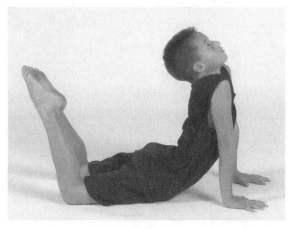

9–15. Modified Lizard for Children

The Modified Lizard for Children addresses the unique concerns of childhood by changing the position of the legs from flat on the floor to bent upward. During a child's growth spurt, primarily from ages 10 to 15, the skeletal structure grows faster than the musculature. The disproportionate length of the muscles impose painfully on the joints they move. While growing pains are natural, they can be eradicated. This TM counteracts the discomfort of the growth spurt by stretching the musculature. This forces muscles to catch up to the growth of the skeleton. The Modified Lizard for Children also targets the quadriceps muscles, which are highly prone to dysfunction in adulthood, and increases the flexibility of the entire pelvic region.

4. Modified Natural Squat for Children

TARGETED AREAS: Pelvic region, knees, and ankles

MODIFIED TARGETED AREAS: Postural control, shoulders, back, and hips

INSTRUCTIONS: Place your feet two inches apart and squat. Straighten your back so that it is perpendicular to the floor. Raise your arms to shoulder height, bend your elbows, and cross your hands behind your head (see 9–16). Keep your heels flat on the floor and your head level so that your chin does not tilt downward or upward. Hold for 30 seconds.

ANALYSIS: If you look at very young children, you will notice that they spend a lot of their time squatting. That is because children are driven by instinct, and squatting is one of the most instinctive positions for the human body. Some children continue to squat until early puberty, albeit at a diminishing rate. The Natural Squat puts children in this healthy and natural position daily, thus promoting the optimal function of their lower back, pelvic region, knees, and ankles. The Modified Natural Squat for Children increases the challenge considerably to make this TM more effective.

Crossing the hands behind the head increases the arms' ability to maintain postural control. The modified arm position also strengthens and stabilizes the entire shoulder girdle. Squatting with a straight spine increases the muscular balance and strength throughout the entire back region. Bringing the legs close together increases the mobility of the hips. Though most adults, except high-performance athletes, would find the Modified Natural Squat for Children too difficult, most kids, with appropriate effort, should be able to maintain this position for the prescribed time. If your child is unable to do so at first, try lowering his or her arms to a neutral position, or curving his or her spine forward, or spreading his or her legs farther apart. Slowly add the

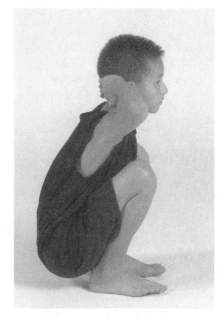

9–16. Modified Natural Squat for Children

modifications back until your child is able to fully express the goal position. The ability to do so is an indication of optimal physical condition that your child will carry with him or her into adulthood.

5. Modified Split for Children

TARGETED AREAS: Lower back, inner thigh muscles, and knees

MODIFIED TARGETED AREAS: Spine, hips, pelvic region, hamstring muscles, and ankles

INSTRUCTIONS: Sit on the edge of a chair or sofa and spread your legs as far apart as you can. Place your heels on the floor and point your toes upward (see 9–17a). Hold for 15 seconds. Next, bend forward and touch the floor as far forward as you can without lifting your buttocks off the seat. Keep your legs straight and your head nestled between your arms (see 9–17b). Hold for 15 seconds.

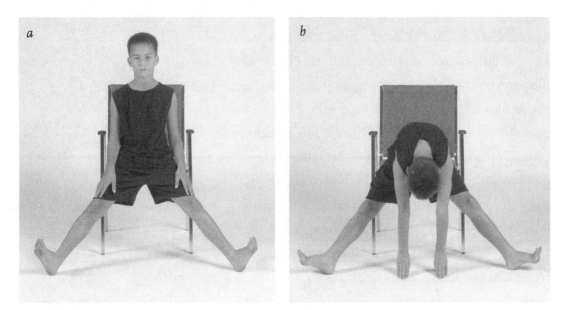

9–17a and b. Modified Split for Children

ANALYSIS: The average child is considerably more flexible than the average adult. This is particularly true in the lower extremities. In my general program, the Split targets the lower portion of the body, including the lower back, by challenging the muscles and joints in these regions to a standing split. But children, much like high-performance athletes, are too flexible for this position. To provide for the biological needs of the lower regions in an appropriate and meaningful way for children, the Split is done while seated.

The Modified Split for Children stretches the inner thigh muscles—which protect and support the knees—without overloading them. The change of position—halfway between my general program and the one for the athletes—also targets the unique concerns of children by taking into account their increased agility. When they bend forward from a raised seated position, their hamstring muscles are restored to their O.M.L., the range of motion at the legs is well maintained, and the mobility of the hips is increased. This TM also takes the spine through its full range of motion, thus lubricating its facet joints with synovial fluid and stretching the paraspinal muscles that run its entire length. Finally, the pointing of the toes stretches the Achilles tendons, which benefits the ankles.

6. Modified Sky Reach for Children

TARGETED AREAS: Spine (specifically, proper postural alignment), shoulders, elbows, wrists, hands, and fingers

MODIFIED TARGETED AREAS: Hips, knees, ankles, and feet

INSTRUCTIONS: Sit comfortably on the floor. Place your left ankle on your right thigh. Then cross your right ankle over your left so that it rests on your left thigh. Curl your toes. Interlace the fingers of your hands and lift your arms up and over your head. With palms facing toward the sky, reach as high as you can (see 9–18). Keep your spine straight. Hold for 30 seconds.

ANALYSIS: Children often develop their musculoskeletal habits by mimicking the adults closest to them. Unfortunately, one of the main things they copy is poor posture, because it is so prevalent among adults. Poor posture, or the improper alignment of the spine, is usually an acquired deficiency that starts in childhood and becomes progressively worse with age. To prevent the physically and psychologically debilitating effects of poor posture in adulthood, children should establish and maintain proper postural control. The Sky Reach reinforces optimal posture by stretching, straightening, and strengthening the muscles most intimately responsible for spinal alignment. This TM also restores the O.M.L. of the rotator cuff muscles, which serve the shoulders, and the forearm muscles, which serve the elbows, wrists, hands, and fingers.

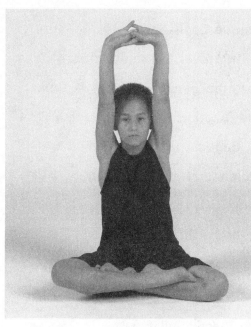

9–18. Modified Sky Reach for Children

The Modified Sky Reach for Children uses the increased flexibility of children to reinforce their optimal level of function. By crossing their legs over each other, the challenge to the hips, knees, and ankles is increased, which increases their rotation and flexibility. The stretch to the exterior muscles of the toes is also intensified in this position. The Modified Sky Reach for Children increases the base level of musculoskeletal function for children so that the inevitable natural reduction of this system through life will be far less than if they had not engaged in this program.

The Modified 3-Minute Maintenance Method: Senior Citizens

Globally, people are living longer than ever before. Unfortunately, they are not necessarily living better. By the time most people reach senior-citizen status at age 65, their joints are riddled with arthritis, their muscles are restricted, and their biomechanical function is highly limited. Seniors are prone to such injuries as falling and breaking bones because they've lost physical coordination and control, and they are unable to participate in many activities because they've lost their ability to move. Eventually they may become dependent on others because they've lost the capacity to manage their own care. This inability to participate in life has very serious consequences. Most senior citizens are generally in great physical pain, have had or need to have joint-replacement surgery, and currently take or have been on some form of pain medication.

Does increased life expectancy have to correspond to a reduced quality of life? Absolutely not. The natural aging process should

Unique Goals and Bonus Benefits

■ **Improves the senior citizen's body mechanics, mobility, and function**

■ **Reduces the likelihood of accidents, trauma, and injury commonly incurred by the elderly**

■ **Stops the cycle of deterioration while counteracting the natural loss of bone density and muscle mass**

result in only a gradual reduction of physical abilities over time. From 30 to 80 years of age, the human body will show a reduction in strength, endurance, and flexibility by approximately 40 percent and a loss of bone density and muscle mass by approximately 30 percent. But aging should not result in a total absence of physical abilities. Although peak musculoskeletal performance diminishes, biomechanical function should remain intact well into the centenarian years. In fact, the grim musculoskeletal conditions that senior citizens face today are consequences not of aging but of years of cumulative musculoskeletal neglect.

Fortunately, musculoskeletal neglect can be counteracted. The Modified 3-Minute Maintenance Method is designed to transform the senior citizen from debilitated to rehabilitated within a year. The program restores a higher level of function and physicality, which arrests the development of further deterioration, by fostering optimal musculoskeletal health in a safe and appropriate way. While severe damage cannot be undone, muscles and joints of any age are remarkably responsive to the provision of their biological needs.

It is important to note that the TMs as pictured do not target elderly people who have stayed fit but rather those who have not. That is why I have provided additional instructions on how to make the TMs progressively more challenging. The goal is to have senior citizens graduate to my general program. Their having done so means they have reclaimed their bodies and, quite possibly, their lives.

1. Modified Bow for Senior Citizens

TARGETED AREAS: Shoulders, elbows, hands, fingers, and knees

MODIFIED TARGETED AREAS: Spine and hips

INSTRUCTIONS: Sit comfortably on the edge of a chair or sofa. Bend over and reach as far as you can with straight arms toward your toes (see 9–19). Spread your fingers wide apart and let your head hang down comfortably so that you are looking at your feet. Hold for 30 seconds. As you progress, you may increase the challenge by placing a thin (1 inch) book under your feet, then a thick (2 to 3 inches) book, then finally, a stool. When you feel that this final stage is easy to perform, you are ready to proceed to this TM in my general program.

ANALYSIS: Years of cumulative musculoskeletal neglect has its biggest effect on the spine. That is why so many senior citizens have poor posture, chronic backaches, and limited mobility. When the components of the anatomy of the spine—the vertebrae, muscles, ligaments, cartilage, and discs—become degraded, they are unable to carry out their intended functions. Indeed, a spine in poor health limits the health of the entire body because it plays an intimate role in almost all movement. Restoring musculoskeletal function must therefore always begin with optimizing the condition of the spine. The Bow targets your spine by taking its joints through their full range of motion and stretching the paraspinal muscles that run its entire length. This is important because it releases the restriction in the vertebrae and in the

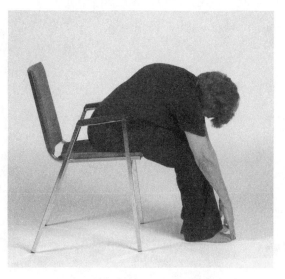

9–19. Modified Bow for Senior Citizens

short, tight musculature of the back. This restriction is responsible for a good deal of pain in the elderly. The Bow also stretches the muscles in your shoulders, elbows, hands, fingers, and knees, relieving further restriction.

To accommodate the senior citizen's bodily limitations, the Bow had to be altered. Getting to the floor and back up again is simply too difficult with the poor physical condition of most seniors. By replicating the TM in a seated position, the Modified Bow for Senior Citizens produces the same benefits—including mobilizing and stretching of your hips—and it does so in a safe and practical way. It also helps to counteract some of the natural loss of bone density and muscle mass (as do all of the following TMs).

As your body allows you to progress, you can increase the challenge as instructed by raising your legs to more closely approximate the TM in my general program. Your ability to meet the increased demand is a sign of advancing musculoskeletal health. As your recovery progresses, you should regain some of the unnatural loss of flexibility, mobility, and endurance you have experienced.

2. Modified Arch for Senior Citizens

TARGETED AREAS: Spine, neck, shoulders, elbows, forearm muscles, wrists, hands, fingers, abdominal muscles, and hips

MODIFIED TARGETED AREAS: Hamstring and calf muscles

INSTRUCTIONS: Stand approximately a foot and a half away from a table with your legs shoulder-width apart. Place your palms flat on the table and spread your fingers wide apart. Slowly lower your head downward while arching your back by moving your pelvis as far away from the table as you can (see 9–20a). Then reverse the movement. Slowly lift your head upward while arching your back in the opposite direction by moving your pelvis as close to the table as you can (see 9–20b). Keep your heels on the floor throughout. This continuous motion should take three seconds. Do this 10 times for a total of 30 seconds. As you progress, you may increase the challenge by

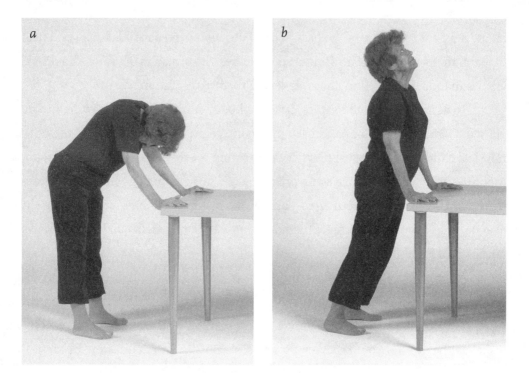

9–20a and b. Modified Arch for Senior Citizens

first placing your hands on a low table, then a chair, and finally on a stool while kneeling on the floor. When you find this final stage easy to perform, you are ready to proceed to this TM in my general program.

ANALYSIS: Arthritis is present in the spinal joints of most senior citizens. This is due to a lifetime of failing to properly mobilize these joints. While arthritic changes often produce the symptoms of limited mobility, stiffness, and pain, they don't have to. Symptoms are the result of continual irritation and dysfunction. By providing for the biological needs of the spine, you eliminate the source of the symptoms, thereby promoting pain-free mobility. You also prevent further deterioration of the structure. The Arch takes the spinal joints through their full range of motion, which lubricates them with synovial fluid. This releases the joints' restriction and provides them with the nourishment they need to function optimally. This TM also stretches and lengthens the short, tight musculature in the neck, shoulders, elbows, wrists, hands, fingers, and hips, all vulnerable areas in the senior citizen.

Moving the position from the floor to a standing position makes the Modified Arch for Senior Citizens less demanding than the Arch in my general program, yet produces the same benefits. This includes the strengthening of your abdominal muscles, which helps to further stabilize your lower back. It also provides a good stretch for your hamstring and calf muscles, helping to restore them toward their O.M.L.

As your body allows you to progress, you can increase the challenge by lowering the surface where you place your hands. Your ability to meet the increased demand is an indication that the flexibility and condition of your spine has significantly improved.

3. Modified Lizard for Senior Citizens

TARGETED AREAS: Spine (specifically, spinal discs), shoulders, elbows, wrists, hands, fingers, and lower back

MODIFIED TARGETED AREAS: Thumbs, calf muscles, ankles, feet, and toes

INSTRUCTIONS: Sit comfortably in a chair or sofa and raise up your feet on their toes. Grasp the top of your pelvis with your thumbs facing forward and your fingers spread across the small of your lower back. Gently push your lower back forward (see 9–21). Lift your chest toward the ceiling and let your head and shoulders follow the lead of the arch, stopping when you see the ceiling directly above you. Hold for 30 seconds. As you progress, you may increase the challenge by sitting on the edge of a chair or sofa, then standing with your back against a wall, and, finally, standing without the support of a wall. When you find this final stage easy to perform, you are ready to proceed to this TM in my general program.

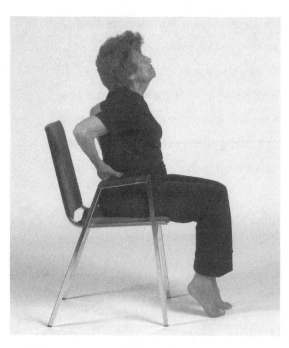

9–21. *Modified Lizard for Senior Citizens*

ANALYSIS: The condition known as a slipped disc is usually not one of the musculoskeletal problems that senior citizens face. By the time most people reach their mid-60s, the contents of the spinal discs are permanently dried up from years of neglect. While this reduces the chances of disc protrusion or herniation, it makes the consequences worse when either does happen. For instance, a slipped disc at 40 may be therapeutically treated since there is still healthy tissue to work with. At 70, a slipped disc usually requires surgery since there is no healthy tissue left. Because surgery at an advanced age is often too dangerous, this can leave the person in pain for the remainder of his or her life. To prevent this condition from occurring, the Lizard pushes the discs back toward their optimal position by stretching the most vulnerable portions of the spine, the lower back. This TM also stretches the muscles that move the shoulder, elbow, and wrist joints.

The Lizard could have been changed from a TM done on the floor to one done in a standing position. However, most seniors have reduced body balance. To make it effective and safe, the Modified Lizard for Senior Citizens is done while seated. The benefits can therefore be extended to your ankles and feet. By getting on your toes, you strengthen your calf muscles and stretch the ankle and toe joints, which counteracts the painful consequences of wearing shoes. This TM also stretches your neck, shoulders, forearms, hands, and fingers, especially the thumbs, thus stabilizing their corresponding joints.

As your body allows you to progress, you can increase the challenge by extending the curve of the arch in your back. Your ability to meet the increased demand is an indication that the spinal discs are in good position and that the range of motion of the spine has been extended. It is also a sign that your balance and physical coordination have been markedly improved.

4. Modified Natural Squat for Senior Citizens

TARGETED AREAS: Lower back, hips, pelvis, knees, and ankles

MODIFIED TARGETED AREAS: Arms (specifically, deltoid, biceps, and fore-arm muscles)

INSTRUCTIONS: Sit comfortably on a chair or sofa and place a stool approximately six inches high under your feet. Lean forward and clasp your shins. Pull your legs in toward your body so that the top of your thighs touch your chest (see 9–22). Hold for 30 seconds. As you progress, you may increase the challenge by using a stool 12 inches high, then 18 inches, and, finally, a chair approximately two feet high. When you find this final stage easy to perform, you are ready to proceed to this TM in my general program.

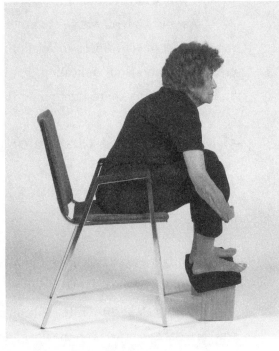

ANALYSIS: There are some cultures with people over 100 who have almost no arthritis and have neither limited mobility nor pain in their lower backs, hips, and knees. This is in sharp contrast to the majority of the global population who suffer from these conditions by the time they reach their 40s. What's their secret? It's that they've

9–22. Modified Natural Squat for Senior Citizens

squatted all their lives. Squatting is a single bodily motion that optimizes the health of a multitude of joints (see targeted areas on page 255). These joints are among the most used, abused, and vulnerable in the body. Their biological needs are also the hardest to provide for: to do so must, in our sitting culture, be purposeful.

Getting into and maintaining the Natural Squat is hard for most people at first and nearly impossible for the average senior citizen. For the latter to get the innumerable benefits from this TM, the position had to be changed. The Modified Natural Squat for Senior Citizens replicates a floor squat by having you bring the knees up to the chest rather than bringing the chest down to the knees. While the benefits are nearly identical to my general program, the method of producing these results is safer, gentler, and more protective. Furthermore, by utilizing your arms to pull your knees up toward your body, you strengthen the muscles of the upper extremities, specifically the biceps and forearm muscles. Finally, this TM is very important for senior citizens because it restores function and health to the targeted muscles and joints—the lower back, hips, pelvis, knees, and ankles—most of which have already incurred much damage and deterioration.

As your body allows you to progress, you can increase the challenge by raising the level of your knees in relation to your chest. Your ability to meet the increased demand is an indication that the muscles are approaching their O.M.L. and that the joints are reaching their full range of motion.

5. Modified Split for Senior Citizens

TARGETED AREAS: Lower back, hips, hamstring and inner thigh muscles, groin region, and knees

MODIFIED TARGETED AREAS: Ankles and feet

INSTRUCTIONS: Sit comfortably on a chair and spread your legs as far apart as you can. Place your heels on the floor and point your toes upward (see 9–23a). Keep your knees slightly bent. Hold this position for 15 seconds. Then bend at your waist

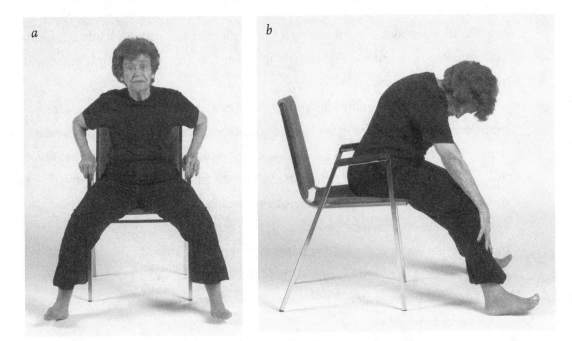

9–23a and b. Modified Split for Senior Citizens

so that you grasp your shins and see the floor (see 9–23b). Hold this position for 15 seconds. As you progress, you may increase the challenge by sitting on the edge of the chair with your knees straight and grasping your shins, then sitting with your knees straight and touching your heels, and, finally, sitting on a low chair or sofa with knees straight and touching the floor. When you find this final stage easy to perform, you are ready to proceed to this TM in my general program.

ANALYSIS: The American Medical Association reports that there will be more than 270,000 total knee replacements and 170,000 artificial hip implants this year alone, mostly performed on older citizens.[2] Why are the knees and hips so vulnerable? Because they bear most of the load and pressure of body weight when moving and sitting, and do so under less than optimal conditions over the course of a lifetime. When the musculature that moves these joints is tight and short, it imposes upon and restricts the joints' movements, which increases their suscep- tibility to wear and tear. In my general program, the Split targets the knees by restoring the O.M.L. of the inner thigh muscles while standing. This TM then targets the hips by taking them through their full range of motion while bending. These positions require a level of balance, coordination, and strength that most seniors do not possess.

By changing the standing position to a seated one the Modified Split for Senior Citizens stretches the inner thigh and groin muscle groups without overburdening the rest of the body. The change of position then facilitates the health of the lower back and hips by bending them. The modifications also add a stretch for the hamstrings, ankles, and feet, thereby providing for their biological needs.

As your body allows you to progress, you can increase the challenge by increasing the width of the split and lowering the bend. Your ability to meet the increased demand is an indication that the targeted muscles can maintain a greater stretch and that the targeted joints can move through a larger portion of their range of motion.

6. Modified Sky Reach for Senior Citizens

TARGETED AREAS: Spine (specifically, proper postural alignment), shoulders, elbows, wrists, hands, and fingers

MODIFIED TARGETED AREAS: Rotator cuff muscles, hips, knees, and ankles

INSTRUCTIONS: Sit on the edge of a chair or sofa and cross your legs at your ankles. Let your knees fall open just past shoulder-width apart. Interlace the fingers of your hands. Keep your spine straight and lift your arms over your head. With palms facing the top of your head and elbows apart, reach as high as you can (see 9–24). Hold for 30 seconds. As you progress, you may increase the challenge by placing your feet on a stool approximately 6 inches, then 12 inches high, and finally on a chair approximately two feet high. When you find this final stage easy to perform, you are ready to proceed to this TM in my general program.

ANALYSIS: Most seniors have exceedingly poor posture because the muscles that maintain proper spinal alignment are too weak to maintain it for long. Poor posture has a devastating effect on both the physiology and psychology of the elderly person. Indeed, I contend that it is poor posture, not circumstance, that contributes most to depression in senior citizens.

The Sky Reach moves you toward the restoration of optimal posture by stretching, straightening, and strengthening the spine. Increasing the length, position, and potency of the spinal muscles corrects acquired postural deviations and makes it possible for you to properly carry yourself through the day. Because of the deficiencies of movement over time, most seniors also have limited function in their shoulders. This TM restores the O.M.L. of the rotator cuff muscles, giving you back more range of motion in the shoulder joints.

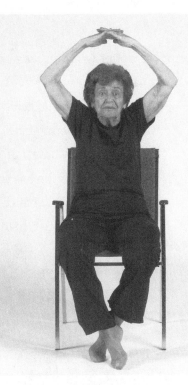

9–24. Modified Sky Reach for Senior Citizens

In most respects, the Modified Sky Reach for Senior Citizens targets the extremities in the same manner as my general program. In fact, the only significant changes are from a position on the floor to a seated one and the placement of the palms. While the modifications result in some loss of benefit to the extremities, this can be minimized by placing a book 3 inches thick under your feet and turning your palms toward the sky. This increases the stretch to the muscles of the elbows, wrists, hands, fingers, hips, knees, and ankles. The modifications do increase the benefit to the lower extremities by externally rotating the hips. This restores the O.M.L. of the internal hip rotator muscles, greatly enhancing the health of these vital joints.

As your body allows you to progress, you can increase the challenge by raising the height of your legs. Your ability to meet the increased demand indicates improvement in the agility and flexibility of your lower extremities.

No matter who you are or what your special physical circumstances, you have the capacity to live a pain-free life. My general program provides the means for the vast majority of people to achieve this, but I didn't want to leave anyone else without a way to realize the same results. If you fall into one of the categories included in this chapter, you now have a program of pain relief and prevention customized for your unique needs. As long as you care for your muscles and joints daily with the Modified 3-Minute Maintenance Method, optimal musculoskeletal health is within your reach. In fact, it's just three minutes away.

Happy Endings: Emily's Story

Emily J., age 14, is an example of a new class of patient. In the past decade, my practice has seen a staggering 75 percent increase in the number of patients under the age of 15. Sadly, this reflects national statistics on the rise of chronic pain in children. Although still thought of as a by-product of aging, musculoskeletal pain is now affecting children as young as five. Emily is healthy, tenacious, and extremely active, but instead of playing with her friends, she found herself in my office, being treated for tendonitis the of pesanserinus in her left knee.

My name is Emily and I am a high school freshman. I have been a cheerleader for five years and captain of the team for the past two years. As a cheerleader, I am required to do running, weight lifting, crunches, jumps, and push-ups at every practice, which is four times a week. Two years ago, I developed a terrible pain in my left knee. When I came home from an uneventful practice hysterically crying, my parents took me to our family doctor. After doing a whole bunch of tests, including X-rays, the doctor said that she didn't know what was wrong with my knee but that it would probably need surgery because it was in bad condition. Although she recommended that I go to an orthopedic surgeon immediately, my parents decided to see if staying off it for a while would help. During this time I could not participate in team practice. Eventually even the slightest things, like going up and down the stairs or walking, became more difficult with every step. I started wearing knee braces and I took Advil every day. None of this worked. I knew this meant surgery, which scared me to death. Then one day it was as if my prayers had been answered. My great-aunt sent me to Dr. Weisberg.

The first thing Dr. Weisberg told me was that if I did what he said to do, I wouldn't need knee surgery. After being told by so many people that I would need it, I thought he was just telling me this to make me feel better. First he gave me specific therapeutic movements to heal my injured knee. (He also told me what was wrong with it, unlike my doctor.) In just two days I felt a lot better. Within a week I was able to walk again, participate in physical education, and go back to cheerleading.

To make sure that my knee and the rest of my body would be protected from anymore injuries, Dr. Weisberg then showed me the Modified 3-Minute Maintenance Method for Children. He told me that if I do his program every day, I can avoid the pain that I see in many of the people around me. He also showed my parents the program for adults. Every morning when my family wakes up, we do it together. Now I don't have to worry about pain anymore. Neither does my dad, who used to have very bad back pain. The program is so easy and quick that it has become a habitual ritual, just like brushing my teeth in the morning. Since I started, I have not taken Advil for my knee. I also have not worn a knee brace. I am able to do everything, still with no pain and no surgery.

10: Planes, Trains, and Automobiles: The Weisberg Way While on the Run

Who it's for: **Anyone**

Where it can be done: **Anywhere**

When it can be done: **Anytime**

I KNOW THAT IT'S OFTEN HARD to find a spare moment to think, let alone to set aside time to optimize the condition of your musculoskeletal system. That's why I created therapeutic movements (TMs) that can be done while you're on the run. You don't need an empty room or special equipment. You don't need a quiet space or privacy. You don't even need to stop what you're doing. The following TMs are designed to work for your body while you're engaged in other work. They are simple, discreet, and won't interfere with or add to your busyness. In fact, they use your busyness as a way to better the quality of your life.

There are four distinct body positions that we place ourselves in over the course of a given day. Together they encompass the total of our daily activities. We *walk* to our cars and around the house and office; we *stand* in line at the grocery store, movies, and bank; we *sit* in front of our computers, in our cars, and around the kitchen table; and we *lie down* when resting and sleeping. Each of these body positions presents an extra chance to perform TMs that provide for the biological needs of your muscles and joints. Each position also has inherent musculoskeletal benefits, such as the positive effect on your hips from walking around the block, and drawbacks, such as the negative effect on your lower back from a long commute on the train, that the TMs can, respectively, enhance and counteract. We will explore the physiological ramifications for each position, how best to transform your daily activity into long-lasting productivity, and why the transformations from the TMs are so complete. I have included three TMs for each distinct position: one for the upper region of the body, one for the mid-region, and one for the lower. You can choose to do one or all of them anytime you want. Each TM takes only 30 seconds to complete. When you consistently take advantage of the opportunities you have to use them, you will significantly raise your level of musculoskeletal health.

Walking

BENEFITS AND DRAWBACKS: Walking is fundamental to the human experience: It is our primary way of moving about. Indeed, the survival of our species depends on it. But the benefits of walking extend far beyond the ability to transport yourself from one place to another. Just as the human body *effects* locomotion, locomotion *affects* the body, and it does so in innumerable ways. Walking enhances the cardiovascular, circulatory, and respiratory systems. It speeds up metabolism, bolsters mental alertness and well-being, and helps prevent many serious illnesses, including diabetes, some cancers, coronary heart disease, and stroke. Most important for our purposes, walking increases bone density and muscle mass and helps to optimize the health of the entire musculoskeletal system.

Walking is the musculoskeletal engagement of your upper, middle, and lower regions while in motion

Walking is a highly complex activity that requires the participation of numerous muscle groups and joints of the body. It also requires sufficient flexibility, coordination, and balance since it is in essence a process of falling and catching up. Here's why: The human body has to fight gravity to vertically maintain itself. Because walking starts with the forward motion of the mid-region of your body, it shifts the center of gravity at your navel to beyond its base of support at your feet. To prevent gravity from pulling you to the ground, your legs catch you by moving forward. This reestablishes the center of gravity over the base of support. Each step then is a departure from and a return to a stable bodily position. This tug of war takes a great deal of effort—far more than you are conscious of—and it is that effort that brings about so many benefits. Because the body diverts building nutrients to the areas most in need, there is a proportional relationship between demand from stress and gravity and total body health. As your body adjusts itself to meet the demands of walking, its condition is elevated and finely tuned.

While there are no drawbacks to walking, it is an activity that can be improved upon. For instance, although walking actively engages your total body, the muscular contractions that build strength and mass in your upper region are substantially less than the contractions in some parts of the lower region. Furthermore, only the joints intimately involved in walking are taken through a range of motion and only partially at that. Finally, a slow pace, poor gait, or postural misalignment can detract from and reduce the benefits of walking. The following TMs are designed to counteract these drawbacks while enhancing the benefits of one of the most natural and perfect therapeutic movements of all.

Upper Region: Walking

INSTRUCTIONS: When you are walking, instead of keeping your arms in a neutral or swinging position, fix them tightly to the sides of your body. Then make fists and squeeze them as hard as you can (see 10–1). Hold this position for six seconds and relax. Do this process five times for a total of 30 seconds.

ANALYSIS: Although walking provides ample opportunity to optimize the health of the upper extremities, they don't receive as much benefit from it as they could because their utilization is limited. This TM targets the musculature in the upper regions of the body by increasing the demand placed upon them. Specifically, the stiffening of the large musculature—the lats, rotator cuffs, and fore-arm muscles—causes them to contract. This iso-metric contraction creates physiological reactions in the musculature that improve circulation, enhance metabolic function, and increase overall strength. The increased demand also helps the region to in-tensify its biomechanical capabilities as the muscles develop and build additional fibers and capillaries to meet the demand. Because the biological needs of these large muscle groups are neglected, the defi-ciency causes innumerable problems; they include the destabilization of the shoulders, elbows, and wrists. This TM gives you an additional way to pro-tect the entire upper region from dysfunction, injury, and pain.

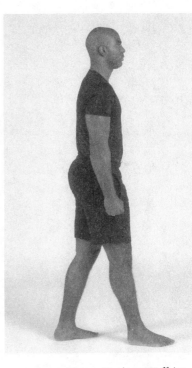

10–1. Upper Region: Walking

Mid-region: Walking

INSTRUCTIONS: While walking, exaggerate the lift of your legs so that your knees are brought to the height of your hips (see 10–2). Do this for a minimum of 30 seconds.

ANALYSIS: The mid-region of the body receives many benefits from walking be-cause it is actively engaged in producing the motion. Nonetheless, these benefits can be significantly improved upon. Ordinarily, your feet clear the ground by ap-proximately one to three inches. Exaggerating the lift brings about many addi-tional musculoskeletal health advantages. First, the increase in demand increases the strength of the musculature responsible for lifting the legs since they must in-crease their abilities to meet the demand. The stronger, more flexible, and more properly balanced the muscles are, the less they impose upon the joints they serve:

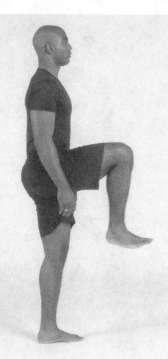

10–2. Mid-region: Walking

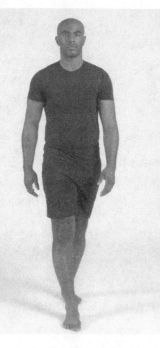

10–3. Lower Region: Walking

the hips and knees. The abdominal muscles are also strengthened because they have to work harder to keep the legs in the air longer. The more powerful your abdomen, the better support and protection it provides for your lower back. Second, the exaggerated motion increases the range of motion in the hip and knee joints, ordinarily minimal in walking. This improves their lubrication and nourishment, thus diminishing their susceptibility to arthritis. Finally, the exaggeration retrains the musculature so that your normal gait becomes higher. This is very important because common injuries caused by stumbling, slipping, and tripping are the direct result of walking with a low gait. By increasing the height of your natural gait, you can prevent these painful and cumulatively debilitating injuries.

Lower Region: Walking

INSTRUCTIONS: While walking, narrow the width of your natural gait by placing one foot directly in front of the other (see 10–3). Keep your line straight by picturing a balance beam beneath your feet. Do this for a minimum of 30 seconds.

ANALYSIS: The lower region of the body receives the most benefit from walking because it produces the action, and it can also be used to provide the most total body benefits while walking. This TM employs the lower region to enhance body balance. Under normal walking conditions, the ability to maintain balance and equilibrium requires the participation and optimal condition of musculature from head to toe. By narrowing the width of your natural gait, you narrow the base of support at your feet. The less support at the feet, the harder it is for your body to maintain balance. As your body fine-tunes itself to meet the increased demand, its agility increases. Improved balance also makes you less clumsy, thus reducing your vulnerability to injury from falls. Finally, the TM increases postural control, coordination, and total core body strength.

Standing

BENEFITS AND DRAWBACKS: Evolution made human beings into bipedal creatures, so our bodies are designed for, and benefit from, standing on two feet. Like walking, standing is a fight against gravity. Specifically, it is a fight to remain erect. As the gravitational forces pull us down, they help to sustain human life by assisting in the flow of fluids to and from our vital organs, maintaining the unique S curvature of our spines, and increasing bone density and muscle mass. Unlike walking, standing is devoid of the benefits of movement. Or is it?

Standing is the musculoskeletal engagement of your upper, middle, and lower regions while stationary.

Standing still does not mean that your body is static. In fact, if you were to watch time-lapse photography of the guards at Buckingham Palace, you would see that even they do not stand completely motionless. That is because when the human body is vertical, gravity causes it to subtly, constantly sway. This swaying in turn causes the center of gravity to shift within its base of support. To prevent falling to the ground, there is a constant interplay between the musculature of the body: the musculature of the lower region contracts to support the vertical load of body weight, the musculature in the mid-region contracts to support the spine, and even some musculature in the upper region contracts to maintain the position of the head. The effect of these contractions is increased strength of total body musculature and increased stabilization of the joints it serves.

But standing has its drawbacks. The constant battle with gravity is a tiring affair. When the musculature responsible for maintaining the vertical position becomes fatigued, it is unable to sustain proper postural control. As postural support wanes, the head and neck droop forward and the upper trunk sinks backward. This slouching position has devastating consequences on body health. (For more on poor posture, see page 190.) Prolonged standing can also slow down circulation, particularly in the lower extremities; place constant pressure upon the spinal joints making them more vulnerable to arthritic changes; and cause some muscles, such as the quadriceps, to shorten and tighten. Fortunately, these drawbacks can be counteracted, and the benefits of standing can be enhanced. Because most of us spend lots of time just standing around—think of how many lines you wait in almost every day of your life—there are plenty of opportunities to take advantage of the following TMs.

Upper Region: Standing

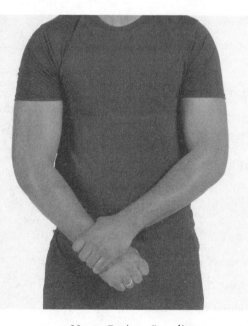

10–4. Upper Region: Standing

INSTRUCTIONS: While standing, bend your elbows slightly and place your left palm on top of your right wrist in front of your abdomen (see 10–4). Try to straighten your right arm while resisting with the left hand. Resist for six seconds and relax. Do this process five times for a total of 30 seconds. Switch hands.

ANALYSIS: As in walking, the upper extremities do not receive much benefit when standing. Yet once again, the time spent in this position presents a golden opportunity to optimize the condition of your upper region. This TM is specifically designed to restore muscular balance in the upper arms. All muscles work in teams of oppositional, complementary pairs to move the joints they serve. These complementary muscles must be well balanced. For the most part, daily living perpetuates the health of the biceps (the front muscles of the upper arms) while neglecting the health of the triceps (the back muscles of the upper arms). When these complementary muscles are imbalanced, they impose on the shoulder and elbow joints, increasing their vulnerability to dysfunction, injury, and pain. This TM strengthens the triceps muscles by isometric contractions so that the balance between them and the biceps muscles is restored. This enhances the condition and function of the entire upper region of the body.

Mid-region: Standing

INSTRUCTIONS: While standing, tighten your abdominal muscles and buttocks as much as you can (see 10–5). Hold for six seconds and relax. Repeat this process five times for a total of 30 seconds.

ANALYSIS: The mid-region of the body—specifically, the lower back—is extremely vulnerable to dysfunction, injury, and pain. This is due in large part to weak abdominal muscles. Abdominal muscles provide the lower back with the majority of its support because they surround two-thirds of the total area. The abdominal wall also protectively encases many vital organs in the region, including the bladder and uterus. Unfortunately, most daily activity does not promote the health of the abdominal muscles, leaving them among the weakest in the body. The consequences are devastating. This

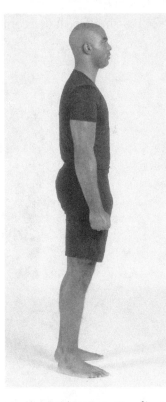

10–5. Mid-region: Standing

TM, which utilizes isometric contractions, provides you with a simple, discreet way to strengthen your abdominal muscles throughout the day. Every time you take advantage of this opportunity, you will produce immeasurable benefits to the midregion of your body. The isometric contraction of the buttocks in conjunction with the abdominal muscles adds additional strength and support to the lower back by optimizing the position of the pelvis. This reduces the fatigue associated with standing and enhances postural control and alignment, which is fundamentally important for total body biomechanical function.

Lower Region: Standing

INSTRUCTIONS: While standing, roll your weight up onto the balls of your feet and toes (see 10–6a). Hold for a moment, then roll your weight back onto your heels (see 10–6b). Repeat in a continuous motion for a minimum of 30 seconds.

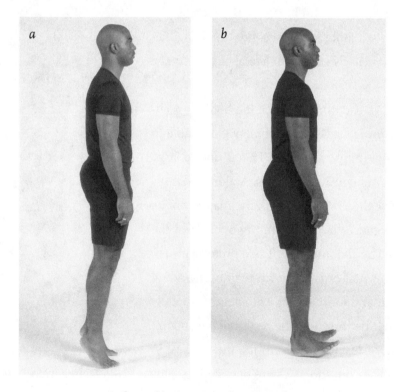

10–6a and b. Lower Region: Standing

ANALYSIS: Standing has its greatest effect, both beneficial and detrimental, on the lower region because it is the body's base of support. As it bears all body weight and maintains balance, the lower region also has to contend with reduced circulation during standing. Gravity takes care of bringing blood to the lower extremities, but standing causes the return circulation back to the heart to slow down. Slowed circulation is a problem: It makes the lower extremities vulnerable to infection, swelling, and deterioration of the veins. It also depletes total body energy since the cardiovascular system has to work harder to compensate for the reduced flow of oxygen.

This TM counteracts the negative effects of standing by activating the musculature and mobilizing the ankle joints. The rolling up and down on the soles of the feet causes a contracting and relaxing of the calf muscles. The interplay between contraction and relaxation increases the return circulation. The more efficient your circulation when you are standing, the less work your cardiovascular system has to do. The effect is increased total body energy. The TM also stretches and strengthens your calf muscles, optimizing their health. Finally, by taking the ankles through their full range of motion, you make them less vulnerable to sprains, strains, and pains.

Sitting

BENEFITS AND DRAWBACKS: Sitting in chairs was born from the need to accomplish time-consuming tasks free of the muscle fatigue that accompanies standing and it does so quite effectively. Sitting rests the lower region of the body while permitting the active use of the middle and upper regions. It demands less from the cardiovascular system, requires less energy to sustain, and encounters less gravitational force. Unfortunately, that is where the benefits of sitting end and its negative physiological effects begin. Sitting is, simply put, the most unnatural and unhealthy of all the possible ways to position the human body. It is, moreover, the most common.

The majority of people spend most of their waking hours sitting. This characteristic of modern culture is so devastating and far-reaching that Chapter 2 is devoted to its consequences. In fact, this entire book can be thought of as a response to the debilitating effects of sitting. Almost all musculoskeletal aches and pains can trace their source to sitting and the sedentary lifestyle it encourages. There are nevertheless some things you can do to make the best of a bad situation. The following TMs are designed to strengthen the areas most weakened by sitting. They also aid in protecting the body and preparing it for this injurious position.

Sitting is the musculoskeletal engagement of your upper and middle region while stationary, as your lower region is at rest.

Because so much of your everyday life is allocated to sitting, you should easily find plenty of opportunities to do these helpful and healing TMs daily. One of the most effective ways to counteract sitting is never to sit for more than 45 minutes at a time. By standing up, walking around, or both at least once every hour, you change your pelvic rotation. This assists in reestablishing the proper curvature of your spine, releasing the short, tight musculature in the hips and lower back, and taking the vertebrae, hips, and knees through at least a partial range of motion. Better still, if you use the time spent sitting—even in a plane, train, or automobile—more productively by doing the following TMs, you will reduce the harmful effects of sitting and make a significant contribution to your musculoskeletal health.

Upper Region: Sitting

INSTRUCTIONS: While sitting, bring your arms up to chest height and bend your elbows so that your hands face each other. Clasp your hands together by interlocking at the midknuckles (see 10–7). Pull your shoulder blades back so that the wing bones in your upper back move closer together. You should feel resistance in the upper regions as well as in your hands. Keep your chin in and your spine straight. Resist the backward pull for six seconds and relax. Do this process five times for a total of 30 seconds. To modify this TM for when you're driving a car, place your hands on opposite sides of the steering wheel. Pull backward with your shoulder blades as explained above.

ANALYSIS: One of the most damaging consequences of sitting is the effect it has on posture. Optimal posture, or the preservation of the unique S curvature of the spine, is fundamental to health because it provides the foundation for almost all bodily functions. Unfortunately, optimal posture is almost impossible to maintain while sitting. Instead, for a variety of reasons, the spine adopts a C curvature, which puts enormous pressure on the vertebrae and discs.

The human body tends to mold itself to the shape of an object it touches. Because most chairs have straight backs, which neither encourage nor support the S curvature of the spine, the midregion stays flush against the backrest while the upper and lower regions bend forward. This creates the C shape mentioned above. Even when a chair provides proper ergonomic support, the upper body still tends to hunch or slouch forward. This is because we reach toward the tasks we are doing with our hands.

Finally, and most important, it is easier and more comfortable to sit with the C curvature because it takes considerable effort and energy to maintain proper posture while seated—more muscular potency than most people possess. To counteract these problems inherent to sitting, you should begin by strengthening your upper back. This TM accomplishes that by isometrically contracting the musculature in the region. The more powerful these muscles become, the more they are able to hold proper postural alignment while you

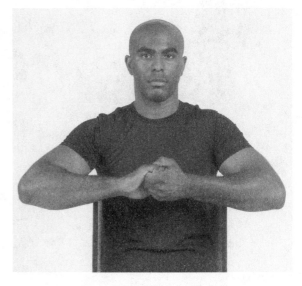

10–7. Upper Region: Sitting

are sitting. This TM also helps to correct some acquired postural deviations, such as rounded shoulders, that you may already exhibit.

Once your upper-back muscles are strong enough, you will be able to make two additional adjustments that will vastly reduce the bad effects of sitting. First, limit the amount of time you lean against a chair's backrest for support. This reduces the likelihood of assuming a C curvature, especially if you are conscious of sitting with a straight spine. Second, bring your tasks to your body instead of bringing your body to your tasks. This reduces hunching forward and considerably extends the life of your spine.

Mid-region: Sitting

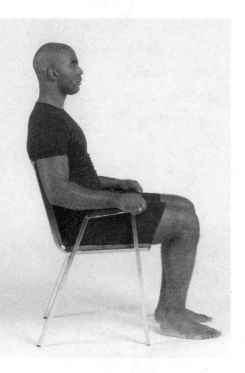

10–8. Mid-region: Sitting

INSTRUCTIONS: While sitting, move your buttocks deep into the chair so that your back is flush against its stationary backrest (see 10–8). Tighten your abdominal muscles and push your whole back against the backrest as hard as you can. Keep your head and neck aligned with the rest of the spine. Hold for six seconds and relax. Do this process five times for a total of 30 seconds.

ANALYSIS: Sitting is responsible for most lower-back pain. This is because the inward curve in the small of your lower back, just below your waistline, is straightened when sitting. Without this critical curvature, the pressure from being partially vertical shifts to areas of the vertebrae, discs, ligaments, and tendons that are unable to bear it without breaking down. Furthermore, because the musculature in the lower back and abdomen remains inactive and unengaged for prolonged periods, sitting weakens it. Without this critical muscular support and protection, the lower back—already the most vulnerable region in the body—falls prey to many painful conditions.

This TM minimizes the risks of sitting by strengthening and balancing the complementary muscle groups of the lower back and abdomen. The additional potency helps to give you better postural control while seated. Stronger lower back and abdominal muscles also help to diffuse the mechanical weight-bearing pressure so that the lower back can better tolerate the straightening of the lumbar curve.

Lower Region: Sitting

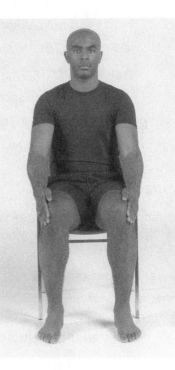

INSTRUCTIONS: While sitting, move your legs to shoulder-width apart and align your heels underneath your knees. Place your hands on the outside of your knees (see 10–9), and try to open your legs while resisting with your hands. Hold for six seconds then relax. Do this process five times for a total of 30 seconds.

ANALYSIS: The previous TMs counteract the bad physiological effects of sitting. In contrast, this TM utilizes the seated position to increase an aspect of physiological health. Specifically, this TM is designed to strengthen the musculature that keeps your pelvic region level when you stand or walk.

Your pelvis is a very vulnerable structure. If the muscles that keep it level are not potent enough, the pelvis will constantly dip out of its proper position. This dipping can cause enormous dysfunction and pain.

10–9. Lower Region: Sitting

The isometric contractions of this TM build up and fine-tune the musculature so that a level pelvis—a vital aspect of optimal standing posture and natural walking gait—is well maintained. The contractions also activate the musculature in the legs, which are otherwise at rest while seated. This increases circulation and prevents cramping in the entire lower region.

Lying Down

BENEFITS AND DRAWBACKS: Lying down gives the body a chance to recuperate from a busy, stressful day. A fully supportive horizontal position provides a necessary reprieve from gravitational forces so that all physiological systems, including musculoskeletal and cardiovascular activity, metabolic and heart rate, and circulation, can slow down. When this occurs, the body is able to replenish the vital resources that have been naturally depleted throughout the day. At least that's what lying down is supposed to do. Unfortunately, most people do not receive even a fraction of these benefits.

Lying down should be a time of rest. However, when most people rest, they aren't really resting. Indeed, without their even realizing it, their bodies are busily contracting their muscles. What causes the body to work hard when it should be taking it easy? Negative psychological states, such as anxiety, worry, and depression, can result in muscular contractions. The inability to properly release this nervous energy accumulates so that by the end of the day the muscular tension has reached its peak. Although you may think that lying down relieves this tension, it doesn't. You actually bring the tension with you into sleep. Sleep itself provides little relief since it is primarily a time for resting the mind, not the musculature. Indeed, considerable musculoskeletal effort is involved in tossing and turning all night, which is why many people complain of waking up tired. Lack of rest affects both your psyche and physiology. It causes you to feel lethargic and overwhelmed and limits the proper function of your muscles and joints. To bring about real rest, you have to learn how to therapeutically relax.

Lying down is the musculoskeletal engagement of your upper, middle, and lower regions while at rest.

Therapeutic relaxation is the opposite of therapeutic movement in that it rids the body of residual muscular contractions rather than causing them to occur. Having spent this entire book encouraging you to move, I now want to leave you with TMs that will enable you *not* to move in the most beneficial way possible.

Upper Region: Lying Down

INSTRUCTIONS: While lying down, tighten the muscles in your face, jaw, neck, shoulders, arms, and hands (see 10–10) for three seconds, then relax. Maintain a normal rate of breathing throughout. Do this process 10 times for a total of 30 seconds. For best results, immediately engage in the following two TMs and then remain lying down for a period of half an hour afterward.

ANALYSIS: See following page.

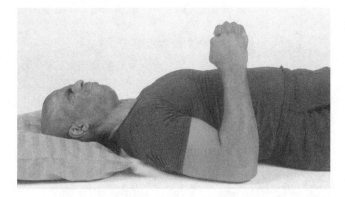

10–10. Upper Region: Lying Down

Mid-region: Lying Down

INSTRUCTIONS: While lying down, tighten the muscles in your chest, back, stomach, hips, and pelvic region (see 10–11) for three seconds and then relax. Maintain a normal rate of breathing throughout. Do this process 10 times for a total of 30 seconds. For best results, perform all three TMs in a row and then remain lying down for a period of half an hour afterward.

ANALYSIS: See following page.

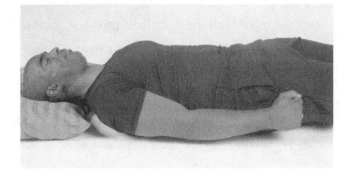

10–11. Mid-region: Lying Down

Lower Region: Lying Down

INSTRUCTIONS: While lying down, tighten the muscles in your thighs, knees, calves, ankles, feet, and toes (see 10–12) for three seconds and relax. Maintain a normal rate of breathing throughout. Do this process 10 times for a total of 30 seconds.

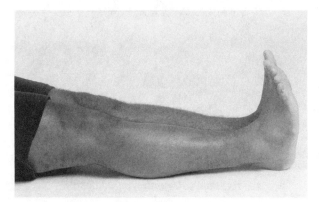

10–12. Lower Region: Lying Down

For best results, perform all three TMs in a row, and then remain lying down for a period of half an hour after you complete this TM.

ANALYSIS: The body and the mind are fundamentally linked. Neither plays a more intimate nor important role than the other in determining total body health, as each deeply affects the other. Just as musculoskeletal conditions influence emotional well-being, emotional conditions influence the function of muscles and joints. This is never more apparent than when it comes to the effects of stress.

Stress, for better or worse, has always been a part of the human experience. It is a survival instinct that initiates both a mental and physical flight-or-fight response. On one hand, stress can be a beneficial tool that inspires creative problem-solving in the face of the challenges and dangers of daily living. On the other hand, stress can be a destructive force that causes a surge in heart rate and blood pressure and suppression of the immune system. Most important for our purposes, stress manifests itself physically in the form of muscular tension. Tension, or the continual contracting of the musculature, leaves you vulnerable to many acute and chronic pains, including headaches, TMJ (from grinding the teeth), stiff neck, sore shoulders, and lower-back pain. It can also cause intestinal problems, ulcers, asthma, infertility, fatigue, and poor posture. These physical problems, in turn, affect the mind by increasing levels of anxiety and depression. In short, stress begets stress.

Because today's world is filled with enormous pressures, many people incorporate psychological stress-reduction techniques into their lives. While many of these techniques recognize the link between the mind and the body, they do not always integrate this connection into their practices. To rid the body of stress, a bridge must be built between the two.

Therapeutic relaxation is a learned skill. It releases the hidden residual tension that lives deep in the memory of your muscle fibers by making a physical appeal to the mind. Here's how it works: There is a biofeedback mechanism between your muscles and your mind. When you intentionally tighten your muscles, your brain detects and recognizes the sensation of tension. When you then intentionally relax the muscules, the brain detects and recognizes the sensation of relaxation. The repetition of contraction and relaxation causes the brain to keenly recognize the distinction between the two muscular positions. By ending with relaxation, you send a message to the brain that the relaxed muscular position is the intended one. The brain responds by sending electrical impulses to the muscles that cause them to relax.

This highly effective process works in reverse too. As muscular activity expressed as tension subsides, so too does the brain activity that causes tension, because the amount of electrical stimulation to the brain is reduced proportionally to the reduction of muscular contractions. Thus the release of physical stress relaxes and calms the mind.

Therapeutic relaxation is also progressive in that the more often you do it, the more fine-tuned relaxation becomes. This means that your mind and body carry with them the ability to respond more appropriately to stress throughout the day. While you cannot avoid the turbulence of living, you can release its effects more efficiently with these TMs so that you can lead a happier, healthier, and pain-free life.

Happy Endings: Carol's Story

Carol R. is a 60-year-old woman who has never had any major injuries, traumas, or diseases. Nonetheless, she spent much of her adult life with chronic pain in her shoulders and neck. At first her pain was low grade and manageable. Like so many of my patients, she had ignored her symptoms, hoping they would just go away. Eventually they always did. But after many years of her suffering like this, the bouts of pain became increasingly longer and the time between the bouts became shorter. By the time she came to see me, her condition had significantly worsened. I diagnosed her as having tendinitis and bursitis of the shoulders, and rotator cuff spasms caused by daily wear and tear.

I've always been one of the busiest women in the world. I am a retired elementary schoolteacher, and I had the blessing of raising four beautiful children. During the early years of their growth, each child participated in specialized sports programs. I acted as chauffeur, cook, cheerleader, and psychologist. Every day I carried on my shoulders everything from food packages and water containers to VCR equipment and cameras. I even carried their hopes, dreams, frustrations, and disappointments. It's no wonder that over the years I developed aches in both of my shoulder blades and my neck. Not having even a minute to spare for myself, I ignored the aches until they turned into constant pain.

A good friend of mine suggested that I see a miracle worker named Dr. Weisberg. When I finally did make the appointment, I immediately explained to him that I had absolutely no time for treatments or exercise programs. Dr. Weisberg told me that my pain was a result of neglect and abuse and that during my busy life I could work on my problematic shoulders and neck. He taught me simple therapeutic movements that I can do while behind the wheel of my car, on the soccer field, in line at the grocery store, at my desk paying bills, and even in front of the stove in my kitchen.

I must admit that when Dr. Weisberg first told me that I could get rid of my pain and *keep it away for good* as long as I made a little time to care for it on a daily basis, I had to laugh. It wasn't that I didn't believe him. Time was simply something that I didn't have much of! As it turned out, I didn't need much. Even people with very hectic schedules like mine can find some *moments* to do his TMs. Lo and behold there were more of those moments than I had first thought. Every chance I got, I did one. It amazed me how simple they were and how discreet. Nobody seemed to notice. Nor did they distract me from the task at hand. I found that I could be busy with my life and my healing at the same time.

The recovery process was amazing. I felt better almost from the beginning and within weeks the pain that had been with me for so long was completely gone. It has been years since those days running around with my young children, but I am as busy as I was then. Today I am a nonprofessional party planner, chocolate maker, and baker. These activities have brought localized stress back to my shoulders and neck. But those simple TMs taught to me by Dr. Weisberg so long ago have given me the freedom to pursue my new interests while keeping my body and spirit free of pain.

Notes

CHAPTER 1

1. The Brain Foundation of Australia, Professor Robert Ouvier, Department of Neurology, New Children's Hospital, March 27, 2003.

2. Hani Raoul Khouzam, "Chronic Pain and Its Management in Primary Care," *Southern Medical Journal*, 2000, 93(10): 946–52.

3. Claudia Kalb, "The Great Back Pain Debate," *Newsweek*, April 26, 2004.

4. Medical Data International, Market and Technology Reports, U.S. Markets for Pain Management Products, Report RP-821922, June 1999; National Institute of Health, "The NIH Guide: New Directions in Pain Research I," Washington, D.C.: GPO, 1998.

5. Chronic Pain Solutions newspaper and website, 2002.

6. American Council for Headache Education, 2004.

7. Reva C. Lawrence et al., "Estimates of the Prevalence of Arthritis and Selected Musculoskeletal Disorders in the United States," *Arthritis & Rheumatism*, vol. 41, no. 5, 778, May 1998.

8. Mark Drangsholt et al., "Temporomandibular Disorder Pain," *Epidemiology*, 203ff.

9. Karen Springen, "Small Patients, Big Pain," *Newsweek*, May 19, 2003.

10. Anne Underwood, "Fibromyalgia: Not All in Your Head," *Newsweek*, May 19, 2003.

11. Chronic Pain Solutions, 2002.

12. Claudia Kalb, "Playing with Pain Killers," *Newsweek,* April 9, 2001.

13. Tim Butler, "Migraines: A Target for Health and Productivity Interventions," *Health and Productivity,* March 2003.

14. Kalb, "Playing with Painkillers."

CHAPTER 2

1. Keith Manchester, *The Archaeology of Disease* (West Yorkshire, England: University of Bradford, 1983), 65.

2. Clark Spencer Larsen, *Skeletons in Our Closet* (New Jersey: Princeton University Press, 2000), 7.

3. Galen Cranz, *The Chair: Rethinking Culture, Body, and Design* (New York: W. W. Norton, 1998), 34.

4. Stuart McGill, "Creep Response of the Lumbar Spine to Prolonged Full Flexion," *Clinical Biomechanics,* 1992, 7: 43–46.

5. Galen Cranz, *The Chair,* 97.

6. Dennis Zacharkow, *Posture: Sitting, Standing, Chair Design, and Exercise* (Springfield, Ill.: Charles C. Thomas, 1988), 213.

7. Larsen, *Skeletons in Our Closet,* 22.

8. Ibid.

9. Patricia S. Bridges, "Prehistoric Arthritis in the Americas," *Annual Review of Anthropology,* 1992, 21: 67–91; P. L. Waker and S. E. Hollimon, "Changes in Osteoarthritis Associated with the Development of a Maritime Economy among Southern California Indians," *International Journal of Anthropology,* 1989, 3: 171–83.

10. David T. Felson and Yuqing Zhang, "An Update on the Epidemiology of Knee and Hip Osteoarthritis with a View to Prevention," *Arthritis and Rheumatism,* 1998, 41: 1343–55.

11. Edward Shorter, "Somatization and Chronic Pain in Historic Perspective," *Clinical Orthopedics and Related Research*, 1997, 336: 52–60.

12. Jenny Pynt, Joy Higgs, and Martin Mackey, "Historical Milestones in the Evolution of Lumbar Spinal Postural Health in Seating," *Spine*, 2002, 27: 2180–89.

13. W. H. Fahrni, "Conservative Treatment of Lumbar Disc Degeneration: Our Primary Responsibility," *Orthopedic Clinics of North America*, 1975, 6(1): 93–103.

14. Christopher Wise, "Osteoarthritis," WebMD.com, 2001.

15. W. H. Fahrni and Gordon E. Trueman, "Comparative Radiological Study of the Spines of a Primitive Population with North Americans and Northern Europeans," *Journal of Bone and Surgery*, 1965, 47B: 2–55.

16. Th. Hettinger, "Statistics on Diseases in the Federal Republic of Germany with Particular Reference to Diseases of the Skeletal System," *Ergonomics*, 1985, 28(1): 69–75.

17. B. Mukhopadhyaya, citing Donald Gunn, "Orthopedics in an Unjust World," CATIA Operators Exchange (COE) conference, Baroda, India, 1998.

CHAPTER 3

1. Health and Human Services Secretary Tommy G. Thompson, "Physical Activity Fundamental to Preventing Disease," U.S. Department of Health and Human Services, June 20, 2002.

2. Daniel D. Bikle, Takeshi Sakata, and Bernard P. Halloran, "The Impact of Skeletal Unloading on Bone Formation," *Gravitational and Space Biology Bulletin*, June 2003, 16(2): 45–54.

3. Ibid.

CHAPTER 4

1. National Consumers League, Over-the-Counter Pain Medication Study, survey conducted by Harris Interactive, December 16–29, 2002.

2. David A. Fishbain, "Chronic Opiod Treatment, Addiction and Pseudo-Addiction in Patients with Chronic Pain," *Psychiatric Times,* vol. XX, no. 2, February 2003.

3. Julian Whitaker, "The Dangers of Overusing Pain Relievers," *Health and Healing,* May 1998.

4. G. Singh, "Gastrointestinal Complications of Prescription and Over-the-Counter Nonsteriodal Anti-Inflammatory Drugs: A View from the ARAMIS Database," *American Journal of Therapeutics,* 2000, 7: 115–21.

5. Ibid.

6. Ibid.

7. Dr. David Graham, study for the U.S. Food and Drug Administration, 2004.

8. M. J. Shield, "Anti-Inflammatory Drugs and Their Effects on Chondrocyte Metabolism In Vitro and In Vivo," *European Journal of Rheumatalogical Inflammation,* 1993, 13: 7–16.

9. Christopher Newton, "Benzodiazepine Abuse," eMedicine.com, March 4, 2001.

10. Cherrill Hicks, "Benzodiazepines Can Ruin Lives," *Sunday Express Magazine,* 1999.

11. Claudia Kalb, "Playing with Pain Killers," *Newsweek,* April 9, 2001.

12. Norman S. Miller and Mark S. Gold, "Abuse, Addiction, Tolerance, and Dependence to Benzodiazepines in Medical and Nonmedical Populations," *American Journal of Drug and Alcohol Abuse,* March 1991.

13. National Consumers League, *Over-the-Counter Pain Medication Study,* 2003.

14. Ibid.

15. Ibid.

16. David Joranson, "Trends in Medical Use and Abuse of Opiod Analgesics," *Journal of the American Medical Association,* 2000, 283: 1710–14.

17. Kalb, "Playing with Pain Killers."

18. Ibid.

19. Department of Health and Human Services report, 1999; Stephen F. Grinstead, *Addiction-Free Pain Management Recovery Guide: Managing Pain and Medication in Recovery* (Independence, Mo.: Herald House/Independence Press, 2002).

20. Barbara Starfield, "Medical Errors: A Leading Cause of Death," *Journal of the American Medical Association*, vol. 282, no. 4, July 26, 2000.

21. *Prevention Magazine* survey, 2002.

22. Burton Goldberg et al., *Alternative Medicine: The Definitive Guide*, 2nd ed., (Berkeley, Calif.: Ten Speed Press, June 2002), 252.

23. Elizabeth Frazão, *The American Diet: A Costly Health Problem*, report of the Food and Consumer Economics Division, Economic Research, USDA, 2002.

24. Ibid.

25. National Nutritional Foods Association (NNFA), results of national consumer survey, 2002.

CHAPTER 6

1. Jack D. Hodge, *The Power of Habit: Harnessing the Power to Establish Routines that Guarantee Success in Business and in Life* (Bloomington, Ind.: 1st Books Library, 1984).

2. Christine Gorman and Alice Park, "The Coming Epidemic of Arthritis," *Time Magazine*, December 9, 2002.

3. A. Bandura, "Self-efficacy mechanisms in human agency," *American Psychologist*, 1982, 37: 122–47. R. deCharms, *Personal Causation: The Internal Affective Determinants of Behavior* (New York: Academic Press, 1968). E. Deci and R. Ryan, *Intrinsic Motivation and Self-Determination in Human Behavior* (New York: Plenum Press, 1986). H. Patrick, A. Ryan, and P. Pintrich, "The Differential Impact of Extrinsic and Mastery Goal Orientations of Males' and Females' Self-Regulated Learning," *Learning and Individual Differences*, 1999, 11(2): 153–72. J. Simons, S. Dewitte, and W. Lens, "Wanting to Have vs. Wanting to Be: The Effect of Perceived Instrumentality on Goal Orientation," *British Journal of*

Psychology, 2000, 91(3): 335–51. R. W. White, "Motivation Reconsidered: The Concept of Competence," *Psychological Review,* 1959, 66: 297–333.

4. Karen Springen, "Small Patients, Big Pain," *Newsweek,* May 19, 2003.

5. Gorman and Park, "The Coming Epidemic of Arthritis."

6. Reva C. Lawrence et al., "Estimates of the Prevalence of Arthritis and Selected Musculoskeletal Disorders in the United States," *Arthritis & Rheumatism,* vol. 41, no. 5, 778, May 1998.

7. Mayo Clinic report, 2004.

8. Gorman and Park, "The Coming Epidemic of Arthritis."

CHAPTER 7

1. Arthritis Foundation, www.arthritis.org, 2004; CDC, "Prevalence of Self-Reported Arthritis or Chronic Joint Symptoms Among Adults," United States, 2001, MMWR 2003: 948–50.

CHAPTER 9

1. Karen Springen, "Small Patients, Big Pain," *Newsweek,* May 19, 2003.

2. Christine Gorman and Alice Park, "The Coming Epidemic of Arthritis," *Time Magazine,* December 9, 2002.

Appendix

The 3-Month Tune-Up: Inventory Checklist

Date: _____   Date of next tune-up: _____   Body parts that need corrective treatment:

Jaw: Pass ☐   Fail ☐ _____

Neck:
Right	*Left*
Pass ☐	Pass ☐
Fail ☐	Fail ☐

_____

Shoulders:
Right (up)	*Left (up)*
Pass ☐	Pass ☐
Fail ☐	Fail ☐

_____

Right (down)	*Left (down)*
Pass ☐	Pass ☐
Fail ☐	Fail ☐

_____

Elbows:
Right	*Left*
Pass ☐	Pass ☐
Fail ☐	Fail ☐

_____

Wrists:
Right	*Left*
Pass ☐	Pass ☐
Fail ☐	Fail ☐

_____

Hands and Fingers:
Right (open)	*Left (open)*
Pass ☐	Pass ☐
Fail ☐	Fail ☐

_____

Right (closed)	*Left (closed)*
Pass ☐	Pass ☐
Fail ☐	Fail ☐

Upper Back: Pass ☐   Fail ☐ _____

Lower Back:
Right	*Left*
Pass ☐	Pass ☐
Fail ☐	Fail ☐

_____

Hips:
Right	*Left*
Pass ☐	Pass ☐
Fail ☐	Fail ☐

_____

Knees:
Right	*Left*
Pass ☐	Pass ☐
Fail ☐	Fail ☐

_____

Ankles:
Right	*Left*
Pass ☐	Pass ☐
Fail ☐	Fail ☐

_____

Feet and Toes:
Right	*Left*
Pass ☐	Pass ☐
Fail ☐	Fail ☐

_____

Index

For additional therapeutic movements, customized pain relief programs,
and daily pain prevention tips, please visit our website: www.painfreelives.com.
